The Good Energy CookBook & Diet Plan

365+ Days of Recipes Inspired by Dr. Casey Means to Optimize Your
Health and Boost Your Metabolism

ANGELA HARPER

Copyright 2024

The contents of this book may not be reproduced, duplicated, or transmitted without the written permission of the author or publisher. Under no circumstances shall the publisher, or the author, be held liable or legally responsible for any damages, compensation, or monetary loss due to the information contained in this book. Either directly or indirectly.

Legal notice: This book is copyrighted. This book is for personal use only. You may not modify, distribute, sell, use, quote, or paraphrase any part or content of this book without the consent of the author or publisher.

Disclaimer: This book is intended for informational purposes only. The information in this book is not a substitute for the advice, diagnosis, or treatment of a medical professional. The theories and practices described are based on Dr. Sebi's teachings and the author's research. The author assumes no responsibility for any adverse effects or consequences resulting from the application of the information provided.

TABLE OF CONTENTS

Introduction 7
    Welcome to the World of "Good Energy" 7
    Dr. Casey Means' Contribution to Metabolic Health 8

Chapter 1: Understanding the Lifestyle for Optimal Health 10
    The Connection Between Metabolism and Well-being 10
    Managing Stress and Sleep Quality 11
    The Mind as a Healing Tool 12
    Monitoring and Optimizing Metabolic Health 13
    Signs of Suboptimal Metabolism and How to Recognize Them 15

Chapter 2: Adopting a Lifestyle that Promotes Optimal Metabolism 17
    Lifestyle and Metabolic Health: What Works and What Doesn't 17
    Practical Ways to Modify Lifestyle to Support Metabolism 18
    Principles of Metabolic Nutrition 20
    Foods to Favor and Foods to Avoid 21
    The Role of Macronutrients 23

Chapter 3: The Diet for Optimal Metabolism 25
    Basics of a Diet that Supports Metabolism 25
    Managing Blood Sugar Spikes 26
    How to Personalize Your Diet Based on Individual Needs 27
    Long-term Benefits of Targeted Nutrition 28

RECIPES 30

Energizing Breakfasts 30
    Coffee Chia Pudding with Coconut and Pecans 30
    Green Shakshuka with Spinach and Avocado 31
    Almond Flour Pancakes with Sugar-Free Blueberry Syrup 32
    Avocado Toast with Smoked Salmon and Radishes 33
    Baked Eggs with Kale and Turkey Sausage 34
    Pumpkin Pancakes with Coconut Syrup and Cinnamon 35
    Mango Smoothie Bowl with Chia Seeds and Macadamia Nuts 36
    Almond Flour Muffins with Blueberries and Lemon Zest 37
    Asparagus and Prosciutto Egg Casserole 38
    Sweet Quinoa Bowl with Nuts and Sugar-Free Maple Syrup 39

Nutritious Lunches 40
    Lettuce Wraps with Smoked Turkey, Avocado, and Tahini Sauce 40

Reimagined Cobb Salad with Kale, Eggs, and Turkey Bacon 41

Tomato and Ginger Soup with Avocado Cream 42

Cauliflower 'Rice' Salad with Peas, Carrots, and Almond Sauce 43

Lettuce Tacos with Bison Meat and Cilantro Salsa 44

Cauliflower Rice Bowl with Spicy Shrimp and Lime Sauce 45

Kale Salad with Berries, Nuts, and Honey Vinaigrette 46

Turkey Chili with Black Beans and Avocado 47

Vegetable Skewers with Tahini and Lemon Sauce 48

Tandoori Chicken with Cucumber Salad and Greek Yogurt 49

Lettuce Wraps with Lamb Meatballs and Tzatziki Sauce 50

Chickpea and Avocado Salad with Lime and Cilantro 51

Zoodles (Zucchini Noodles) with Cashew Alfredo Sauce 52

Tuna Salad with Celery, Red Onions, and Greek Yogurt 53

Lettuce Wraps with Hummus, Cucumbers and Kalamata Olives 54

Healthy and Tasty Dinners 55

Roast Chicken with Avocado Chimichurri Sauce 55

Sesame-Crusted Salmon Bowl with Kale and Tamari Soy Sauce 56

Oven-Baked Pork Ribs with Coconut Pineapple BBQ Sauce 57

Nut-Crusted Cod Fillet with Roasted Asparagus 58

Beef and Cauliflower 'Barley' Soup with Roasted Vegetables 59

Turkey Burgers with Guacamole and Baked Sweet Potato Fries 60

Baked Eggplant and Tomato Casserole with Almond Mozzarella 61

Grilled Fish Tacos with Mango Salsa and Cilantro 62

Lamb Stew with Root Vegetables and Rosemary 63

Carrot and Curry Soup with Coconut Milk 64

Salmon Burgers with Dill and Lemon Sauce 65

Roasted Cauliflower with Tahini and Pomegranate 66

Almond Flour Pizza with Prosciutto and Arugula 67

Cauliflower Soup with Ginger and Turmeric 68

Zucchini Meatballs with Marinara Sauce and Vegan Parmesan 69

Metabolism-Friendly Snacks 70

Celery Sticks with Almond Butter and Honey 70

Kale Chips with Smoked Paprika and Sea Salt 71

Cauliflower Popcorn with Olive Oil and Vegan Parmesan 72

Prosciutto Roll-Ups with Almond Cheese and Green Olives 73

Avocado, Spinach, and Green Apple Smoothie 74
Energy Bites with Dates, Cacao, and Nuts 75
Mini Spinach and Mushroom Frittatas 76
Beet Hummus with Vegetable Crudités 77
Toasted Macadamia Nuts with Rosemary and Sea Salt 78
Nori Seaweed Snacks with Avocado and Sesame Seeds 79

Wellness Beverages 80

Matcha Latte with Almond Milk and Honey 80
Iced Lemon Ginger Tea with Fresh Mint 81
Coconut Pineapple Smoothie with Turmeric and Ginger 82
Ginger, Lemon, and Turmeric Herbal Tea 83
Bulletproof Coffee with Coconut Oil and Cinnamon 84
Chilled Almond Milk with Cocoa and Vanilla 85
Iced Hibiscus Tea with Lime and Honey 86
Green Smoothie with Kale, Cucumber, and Green Apple 87
Chilled Golden Milk with Turmeric and Ginger 88
Green Juice with Celery, Spinach, and Apple 89

Guilt-Free Desserts 90

Vegan Lemon Cheesecake with Almond Crust 90
Chocolate Mousse with Avocado and Coconut Syrup 91
Paleo Carrot Cake with Coconut Cream 92
Banana Ice Cream with Pecans and Cacao 93
Almond Flour Brownies with Walnuts 94
Apple Tartlets with Almond Crust and Cinnamon 95
Oatmeal Blueberry Cookies with Coconut Flour 96
Coconut Lime Mousse with Ginger 97
Dark Chocolate Truffles with Chili Pepper 98
Pumpkin Pie with Nut Crust and Maple Syrup 99

Special Occasion Recipes 100

Quinoa Paella with Shrimp and Vegetables 100
Zucchini Lasagna with Vegan Ricotta and Spinach 101
Baked Chicken with Walnut Sauce and Roasted Broccoli 103
Sweet Potato Gnocchi with Mushroom Sage Sauce 104
Lettuce Tacos with Bison Meat and Avocado Salsa 105
Quinoa Paella with Shrimp and Vegetables 106

Chicken Fajitas with Peppers and Cilantro Salsa 108
BONUS WITH QR CODE 109

Introduction

Welcome to the World of "Good Energy"

Stepping into the world of "Good Energy" opens up a gateway to revitalizing your health through the transformative power of metabolic optimization. This journey is not merely about altering what we eat; it encompasses a holistic approach that reverberates through every aspect of our lives, guiding us towards sustained wellness and vitality. When we talk about "Good Energy," we're delving into a state of being that transcends the physical. It's the vibrant spirit you carry through your day, the mental clarity that enhances your interactions, and the emotional stability that underpins your daily experiences. Such a comprehensive form of health is not achieved by chance but through deliberate, informed choices in our lifestyle and nutrition, informed by cutting-edge science and traditional wisdom alike.

The concept of "Good Energy" is rooted in the recognition that our bodies are complex systems, highly responsive to our environment, our diets, and our ways of life. Each choice we make has the potential to either disrupt this system or to foster its proper functioning. Thus, understanding the mechanics of our metabolism becomes not just a scientific endeavor, but a personal one. Metabolism, at its core, is the entirety of biochemical processes that occur within our bodies to maintain life. It's how our cells convert the food we eat into the energy we need to function from day to day. However, this is not just about energy in the form of calories but energy that is efficient, clean, and harmonizing with our bodies' needs. When our metabolism works optimally, we feel it as a surge of "Good Energy"—energy that lasts, that empowers, and that rejuvenates.

Unfortunately, many of us navigate through life feeling less than our best. We accept fatigue, brain fog, and emotional instability as par for the course, symptoms of busy lives and aging. Yet, what if these common ailments are actually indicators of suboptimal metabolic health? What if the lethargy and the overwhelming sense of weariness are not inevitable? This is where the shift towards "Good Energy" begins—by listening to our bodies and responding with choices that support metabolic enhancement.

The journey to "Good Energy" is personalized. It acknowledges that each person's body is unique, with its own strengths and vulnerabilities. Therefore, the path to optimizing your metabolic health is not about following a one-size-fits-all diet or lifestyle. Instead, it's about understanding the principles that govern good metabolic health and adapting them to fit your individual circumstances. It involves learning how to listen to your body's signals and respond appropriately with nutritional choices, sleep patterns, stress management techniques, and more. For instance, consider the impact of refined sugars and processed foods on our metabolism. These foods can cause spikes in our blood sugar levels and lead to fluctuations in our energy, affecting our mood and cognitive functions. By choosing whole, unprocessed foods, we can maintain more stable blood sugar levels, which supports sustained energy and overall well-being. Moreover, "Good Energy" is not achieved in isolation. It is nurtured through community, through sharing meals and wellness practices, and through supporting each other in our individual journeys toward better health. It's about building environments—both at home and in our wider communities—that foster healthy choices and make them accessible and enjoyable.

As we embark on this journey together through the pages of this book, we will explore how to harness the principles of metabolic health to not only improve our physical health but also enhance our mental and emotional well-being. The goal is to equip you with the knowledge and tools to transform your life by transforming your energy. This isn't just about living longer—it's about living better, with more vitality, more resilience, and more "Good Energy" to enjoy every moment of our lives. Embrace this journey as an opportunity to rediscover your innate potential for health and happiness. Let "Good Energy" be your guide to a life of enhanced health, deeper satisfaction, and profound well-being. Welcome aboard, let's illuminate the path to your best self together.

Dr. Casey Means' Contribution to Metabolic Health

In the rapidly evolving field of metabolic health, few names have emerged as prominently and influentially as Dr. Casey Means. A Stanford-trained physician, Dr. Means has carved a unique niche in the intersection of technology, nutrition, and preventive medicine, propelling a paradigm shift in how we understand and manage our metabolic health. Her contributions have not only enhanced the scientific community's understanding but have also made a profound impact on everyday lives, guiding individuals toward a more informed and proactive approach to their health. Dr. Means' journey into metabolic health was spurred by her observations of the limitations within traditional medical practice, particularly in addressing chronic conditions. She noticed a common thread among many ailments: a foundational disturbance in metabolic processes. This insight led her to delve deeper into metabolic health, eventually advocating for a shift from reactive medicine to a more preventive, holistic approach. Her philosophy centers on the belief that understanding and optimizing metabolic function is key to preventing disease and enhancing overall wellness.

One of Dr. Means' significant contributions is her emphasis on the role of glucose management in metabolic health. Through her research and public engagements, she has elucidated how fluctuations in blood glucose levels can have far-reaching effects on our energy levels, mood, cognitive function, and long-term health. Her work has highlighted how modern diets, rich in processed foods and sugars, directly contribute to metabolic disruptions, leading to a host of health issues from diabetes to heart disease and beyond. Dr. Means advocates for the use of continuous glucose monitoring (CGM) technology as a tool for real-time, personalized insights into one's metabolic health. By understanding how different foods and lifestyle choices affect glucose levels, individuals can make more informed decisions that support their unique metabolic needs. This application of technology in everyday health management represents a significant leap forward in personalized medicine, making Dr. Means a pioneer in integrating tech solutions with health practices.

Moreover, Dr. Means has been instrumental in popularizing the concept of metabolic flexibility—the ability of an organism to adapt fuel oxidation to fuel availability. This concept has profound implications for weight management, energy utilization, and overall health resilience. By promoting diets and lifestyles that enhance metabolic flexibility, she has helped countless individuals regain control of their health, improving their quality of life and reducing their risk of chronic disease. Beyond her clinical and technological innovations, Dr. Means has also been a vocal advocate for systemic changes in how we approach food and health policies. She argues that a shift towards whole, nutrient-dense foods and away from sugar-laden, processed options is crucial for public health. Her advocacy extends into the realms of education, where she pushes for greater awareness of nutritional science in schools, and public policy, where she supports initiatives that promote healthy food environments. Dr. Means' educational efforts extend through her prolific writing and speaking engagements, where she has the ability to translate complex scientific concepts into accessible, actionable advice. Her articles and talks are rich with practical tips, backed by rigorous science, yet conveyed with the clarity and warmth that encourage positive change. Her voice is a beacon for those looking to navigate the often confusing landscape of health information, providing clarity and hope. Her influence is also evident in her collaborative efforts with other health professionals and organizations. By fostering a community of like-minded experts, she has helped build a broader, integrative approach to health care that prioritizes patient empowerment and preventive care over the traditional symptom-management model.

In essence, Dr. Casey Means' contribution to metabolic health is profound and multifaceted. Her work not only advances scientific understanding but also transforms lives by equipping individuals with the knowledge and tools necessary for maintaining optimal health. As we explore the principles of "Good Energy" in this book, Dr. Means' insights and methodologies will be a recurring theme, guiding us through the practical applications of her pioneering work. Her legacy is not just in her research and innovations but in the everyday victories of those who have taken her lessons to heart, transforming their health trajectories toward a brighter, more vibrant future.

Chapter 1: Understanding the Lifestyle for Optimal Health

The Connection Between Metabolism and Well-being

Understanding the integral relationship between metabolism and well-being is pivotal in navigating the complexities of modern health. Metabolism, often simplified to the body's method of converting food into energy, is far more intricate and influences more than just our physical vigor; it is the bedrock of our overall well-being, affecting mental health, emotional balance, and even social interactions.

At its essence, metabolism dictates the rate and efficiency with which our bodies utilize nutrients. This biochemical process not only powers physical activities but also regulates hormonal balances, repairs cellular damage, and supports cognitive functions. When our metabolic processes function optimally, they foster an environment where energy levels are sustained, mental clarity is enhanced, and bodily systems operate in harmonious synchrony. However, when these processes falter, the effects resonate beyond mere physical fatigue, potentially leading to mood fluctuations, impaired cognitive abilities, and a general decline in quality of life. The state of our metabolism is inherently tied to our lifestyle choices—from the foods we consume to our physical activity levels and even the amount of sleep we get. Each of these factors plays a crucial role in either supporting or undermining metabolic health. For instance, diets high in processed sugars and unhealthy fats can impede metabolic efficiency, leading to increased fat storage, higher levels of inflammation, and elevated blood sugar levels. This can manifest not only in weight gain but also in a diminished mental state and lower energy levels. Conversely, a diet rich in nutrients, fiber, and appropriate proteins supports the myriad enzymatic reactions that constitute healthy metabolism. Foods such as leafy greens, whole grains, and lean proteins can enhance metabolic pathways that are essential for energy production and efficient cellular function. Beyond nutrition, physical activity is another cornerstone of metabolic health. Regular exercise boosts the body's metabolic rate, which helps in burning calories more efficiently even during periods of rest. It also stimulates the release of hormones that promote a sense of well-being, further linking physical health with emotional and mental states.

The impact of metabolic health extends into the psychological realm. A well-maintained metabolism supports the production and regulation of neurotransmitters such as serotonin and dopamine, which are crucial for mood stabilization and the promotion of feelings of happiness and well-being. An imbalance in these biochemicals often correlates with mood disorders such as depression and anxiety, illustrating a direct link between metabolic health and mental health. Moreover, the influence of metabolic health is not confined to the individual. It plays a significant role in social interactions and public health at large. Individuals with optimal metabolic function tend to have more energy and a more positive outlook on life, which are contagious traits that can improve the well-being of their communities. Conversely, the strain of metabolic diseases such as diabetes and obesity not only affects individuals but also places a significant burden on healthcare systems and economic structures. Addressing metabolic health, therefore, requires a holistic approach that encompasses diet, exercise, sleep, and stress management—all of which interlink to form a comprehensive picture of our health. By understanding these connections, individuals can make more informed decisions about their lifestyles, leading to improved metabolic function and, consequently, enhanced overall well-being.

As we delve deeper into the connection between metabolism and well-being, it becomes evident that our bodily health is not merely a function of what we eat or how much we exercise, but a complex interplay of various lifestyle choices. Embracing a lifestyle that promotes metabolic efficiency is not just about enhancing physical health but is a vital step towards achieving a richer, more vibrant life. Through this holistic lens, we see that our daily choices are not just shaping our physical bodies but are fundamentally defining the quality of our lives and our interactions with the world around us.

Managing Stress and Sleep Quality

In the quest for optimal health, the significance of managing stress and ensuring quality sleep cannot be overstated. These elements of health are not only fundamental in maintaining metabolic balance but are also critical in achieving a life filled with vigor and tranquility. This relationship is cyclical: while effective stress management can improve sleep quality, good sleep can profoundly mitigate the impacts of stress on our bodies and minds, creating a foundation for a more resilient and energetic self.

Stress, in its essence, is the body's natural response to challenges and pressures, whether they stem from work, relationships, or other life circumstances. While a certain level of stress can be motivating and lead to enhanced performance, chronic stress has the opposite effect, deteriorating one's health profoundly. When stress becomes a constant companion, it can disrupt nearly every system in the body. It can suppress the immune system, increase the risk of heart attack and stroke, and contribute to conditions like obesity and depression. Understanding how to manage stress is thus not merely about enhancing emotional well-being but about safeguarding physical health. One of the most direct impacts of stress is on the metabolic system. Under stress, the body produces increased levels of cortisol, a hormone that is useful in short bursts but harmful when elevated long-term. High cortisol levels can lead to various metabolic issues, including weight gain, increased blood pressure, and disruption of blood sugar levels, all of which undermine metabolic health. Managing stress, therefore, becomes a crucial component of maintaining metabolic balance and ensuring the body's energy systems function optimally.

Turning to sleep, it is well-documented that quality sleep is a cornerstone of good health. While we rest, our bodies undergo numerous processes essential for physical and mental recovery. Sleep affects almost every type of tissue and system in the body – from the brain, heart, and lungs to metabolism, immune function, mood, and disease resistance. A continuous lack of sleep or poor-quality sleep increases the risk of high blood pressure, cardiovascular disease, diabetes, depression, and obesity. Quality sleep acts as a moderator for the body's metabolic processes. During sleep, important hormones are released, including those that help regulate energy metabolism. Sleep supports healthy growth hormone levels, which plays a part in how our body uses energy and maintains muscle and tissue health. Inadequate sleep can alter hormone production, including insulin. Insulin controls our blood glucose level; thus, disrupted insulin production due to poor sleep can lead to higher blood sugar levels, which, over time, may increase the risk of type 2 diabetes. Managing stress and improving sleep quality are intertwined challenges that require integrated solutions. Effective stress management involves a variety of techniques and lifestyle adjustments.

Mindfulness meditation, for instance, has shown significant benefits in reducing stress. This practice involves sitting quietly and paying attention to thoughts, sounds, the sensations of breathing, or parts of the body, bringing your mind's attention to the present without drifting into concerns about the past or future. This approach helps enhance emotional resilience and reduces reactivity to distressing situations.

Exercise is another powerful tool for stress reduction. Physical activity increases the production of endorphins, the brain's feel-good neurotransmitters, and in doing so, not only minimizes the ill effects of stress but also enhances overall mood. Regular physical activity can also improve the quality of sleep, not only helping you fall asleep faster but also deepening your sleep. Sleep hygiene is critical for improving sleep quality. This includes maintaining a consistent sleep schedule, creating a bedtime routine that signals to your brain that it's time to wind down, and optimizing your bedroom environment – ensuring it is dark, quiet, and cool. Avoiding stimulants such as caffeine and electronic devices before bedtime can also promote deeper, more restorative sleep. Nutrition also plays a key role in both stress management and sleep quality. Diets rich in magnesium, omega-3 fatty acids, and B vitamins have been shown to reduce the effects of stress on the body. Likewise, consuming foods that promote sleep, including those rich in tryptophan, magnesium, and melatonin, like dairy products, nuts, and cherries, can assist in achieving a more restful night.

In conclusion, managing stress and sleep quality are not isolated health strategies but are deeply interconnected. By addressing these areas comprehensively, individuals can not only improve their metabolic health but can also enhance their overall quality of life, making these practices essential components of a lifestyle geared towards optimal health.

The Mind as a Healing Tool

The concept that the mind can act as a potent instrument in healing and health maintenance is not merely an idea rooted in spiritual or new-age thought, but a well-supported notion in modern medical and psychological research. The role of cognitive and emotional factors in physical health is profound and multifaceted, influencing everything from the immune response to hormonal balance and metabolic processes. Embracing the mind as a healing tool offers a transformative approach to health, one that harnesses the interconnectivity of mental and physical well-being to foster resilience, recovery, and longevity.

Understanding how the mind can influence physical health begins with the concept of the "mind-body connection." This term encompasses the biochemical, neural, and hormonal channels through which cognitive and emotional stimuli can affect bodily functions. The central nervous system, particularly the brain, plays a crucial role in interpreting thoughts and emotions, which in turn can dictate bodily responses. For instance, chronic stress can lead to prolonged secretion of cortisol, which affects the body detrimentally in several ways– increasing glucose levels, suppressing immune function, and disrupting sleep, among other effects. Conversely, positive mental states such as joy, contentment, and peace can induce beneficial physiological responses. These states are associated with the production of health-promoting hormones like endorphins and serotonin, which not only improve mood but also enhance immune function and promote metabolic health. Recognizing the power of the mind in health means understanding that our thoughts, attitudes, and emotions significantly impact our overall well-being. One of the most direct ways in which the mind can be harnessed as a healing tool is through the practice of mindfulness. Mindfulness involves maintaining a moment-by-moment awareness of our thoughts, feelings, bodily sensations, and surrounding environment. This practice is often cultivated through meditation, which has been shown to reduce stress, anxiety, and depression. Moreover, mindfulness meditation has been found to improve symptoms of various physical conditions such as irritable bowel syndrome, fibromyalgia, and psoriasis, by moderating stress responses and enhancing immune function. Cognitive-behavioral therapy (CBT) is another powerful modality where the mind's healing capabilities are leveraged to treat a range of health issues. CBT works by changing negative thought patterns that contribute to and exacerbate emotional difficulties and dysfunctional behaviors. This therapy is particularly effective in treating depression, anxiety, and eating disorders, which can all have profound effects on physical health. By addressing the mental components of these conditions, CBT can indirectly improve physical health outcomes. Visualization and guided imagery are techniques that involve focusing and directing the imagination toward positive visualizations of wellness and health. Athletes often use these techniques to enhance performance, which is a testament to their efficacy. In medical settings, guided imagery can reduce pre-surgery anxiety, enhance postoperative recovery, and even help in managing chronic conditions such as asthma and chronic pain.

The healing power of the mind is also evident in its impact on the placebo effect—an excellent example of how expectation and belief can physically alter the body's chemistry. Studies have shown that when people believe they are receiving a treatment that will benefit them, often they experience physiological benefits even if the treatment is inert. This phenomenon highlights the mind's capacity to influence physical health in substantial, measurable ways. Social connection and emotional expression constitute another crucial aspect of how the mind can influence health. Relationships and social interactions can have significant health implications. Positive relationships, characterized by support and understanding, can boost mental health, which in turn impacts physical health. Conversely, isolation and poor social relationships are linked with an increased risk of mortality comparable to well-established risk factors such as smoking. In sum, embracing the mind as a healing tool involves recognizing the substantial influence that our mental and emotional states exert on our physical health. It encourages an integrated approach to health care that addresses the psychological, social, and behavioral aspects of wellness. By cultivating mental resilience and emotional well-being, we do not just improve our mental health; we lay the groundwork for a healthier, more vibrant life. This holistic view, acknowledging the profound synergy between mind and body, equips us with a more complete understanding of what it means to live healthily. In this way, the mind is not only recognized as a mirror reflecting our physical health but as a powerful agent capable of shaping it.

Monitoring and Optimizing Metabolic Health

Metabolic health is a cornerstone of overall wellness, affecting everything from energy levels and weight to mood and long-term disease risk. Monitoring and optimizing one's metabolic health is therefore not merely a matter of preventing illness but is integral to fostering a life of vitality and longevity. This complex process involves a careful blend of observation, intervention, and lifestyle adaptation to ensure that all bodily systems are functioning at their peak. Understanding metabolic health begins with recognizing its foundational components: glucose control, lipid levels, blood pressure, body composition, and hormonal balance. Each of these factors plays a critical role in how efficiently and effectively the body converts food into energy, repairs tissue, and regulates vital functions. However, achieving and maintaining optimal metabolic health goes beyond merely avoiding sickness—it's about fine-tuning the body's systems to operate at their best. To monitor metabolic health effectively, one must first establish a baseline of key biomarkers. These typically include blood glucose levels, cholesterol profiles, blood pressure readings, body fat percentage, and various hormone levels. Regular tracking of these indicators provides invaluable insights into how well the metabolic system is functioning and can signal early disturbances that might not yet have manifested as symptoms. This proactive approach allows individuals to make informed decisions about their health before issues become entrenched. Advancements in technology have significantly enhanced our ability to monitor these biomarkers. Wearable devices that track physical activity and sleep patterns, apps that help log dietary intake, and home testing kits for blood sugar and cholesterol are just a few examples of how modern tools can aid in maintaining metabolic health. Furthermore, continuous glucose monitors (CGMs) offer a real-time look at how different foods affect blood sugar levels, providing a personalized approach to managing diet and preventing glucose spikes that can lead to insulin resistance.

Optimizing metabolic health involves more than just monitoring; it requires an active engagement in modifying lifestyle habits based on the data collected. Diet plays a crucial role in this process. Consuming a balanced diet rich in whole foods—such as vegetables, fruits, lean proteins, and healthy fats—supports metabolic functions and prevents the common pitfalls of excessive sugar and processed food consumption. This dietary approach helps stabilize blood sugar levels, reduces inflammation, and supports healthy weight management. Physical activity is another pillar of metabolic health. Regular exercise not only helps burn calories and build muscle but also improves insulin sensitivity, enhances cardiovascular health, and boosts mood through the release of endorphins. The type, duration, and intensity of exercise will vary from person to person, but the consistent inclusion of physical activity is essential for optimizing metabolic functions. Sleep must not be overlooked in the quest for metabolic optimization. Quality sleep is crucial for the body's healing processes, including the repair of cellular damage and the balancing of hormones that regulate appetite and stress. Ensuring seven to nine hours of uninterrupted sleep per night can significantly impact metabolic health, influencing everything from mood and cognitive function to weight and energy levels.

Stress management also plays a significant role in maintaining metabolic balance. Chronic stress can lead to a host of metabolic issues, including high cortisol levels, poor sleep quality, and uncontrolled blood sugar spikes. Techniques such as mindfulness meditation, yoga, and regular relaxation can help mitigate the effects of stress and promote a more balanced metabolic state. Regular medical check-ups and consultations with healthcare professionals can provide additional insights and guidance on optimizing metabolic health. Medical experts can offer tailored advice and interventions based on individual health profiles, family history, and personal goals. This professional input is crucial in navigating the complexities of metabolic health, ensuring that individual strategies are both effective and sustainable.

In conclusion, monitoring and optimizing metabolic health is a dynamic and continuous process that requires a comprehensive approach, integrating diet, exercise, sleep, and stress management. By taking control of these aspects with the support of modern technology and professional advice, individuals can enhance their metabolic functioning, leading to improved health outcomes and a higher quality of life. This proactive stance empowers people to not just live longer but to live better, with more energy, resilience, and vitality in every aspect of life.

Signs of Suboptimal Metabolism and How to Recognize Them

Recognizing the signs of suboptimal metabolism is crucial in taking early steps toward improving one's metabolic health, a vital component of overall wellness. A well-functioning metabolism not only aids in maintaining an ideal weight but also ensures that the body efficiently processes nutrients, maintains energy levels, supports brain function, and regulates hormonal balance. When metabolism is not functioning optimally, it can manifest in various physical, emotional, and mental symptoms that can significantly reduce the quality of life. By understanding these signs, individuals can take proactive measures to address underlying issues before they evolve into more serious health conditions. One of the most evident signs of suboptimal metabolism is unexplained weight changes. This includes both unexpected weight gain and difficulty in losing weight despite maintaining a healthy diet and regular exercise. When the metabolism slows down, the body may become less efficient at burning calories, leading to fat accumulation. On the other hand, an unexpectedly rapid weight loss can also signify metabolic distress, potentially pointing to conditions such as hyperthyroidism, where the metabolism runs too quickly. Another critical indicator is persistent fatigue. If you are experiencing constant tiredness despite getting adequate sleep, it could be a sign that your metabolic processes are not producing enough energy to meet your body's needs. This type of fatigue often feels overwhelming and isn't relieved by sleep, indicating that the body's energy production is compromised, possibly due to imbalanced hormone levels or dysfunctional mitochondrial activity.

Fluctuations in blood sugar levels are also a telltale sign of metabolic issues. Symptoms such as hunger pangs soon after eating, irritability or lightheadedness between meals, or sudden energy crashes can all suggest that the body is not properly regulating glucose levels. These signs point towards insulin resistance, a common metabolic problem where cells fail to respond normally to insulin, preventing glucose from entering the cells and leading to high blood sugar levels. Digestive issues can also be reflective of metabolic health. Frequent bloating, gas, constipation, or diarrhea can indicate that the body is not effectively metabolizing and absorbing nutrients. Poor gut health can lead to an impaired metabolism as the digestive system plays a significant role in hormone production, including those involved in hunger regulation and energy balance. Changes in mood and mental health are often overlooked as signs of metabolic imbalance but are profoundly connected. Conditions such as depression, anxiety, and mood swings can be exacerbated by poor metabolic health. A poorly functioning metabolism can affect the brain's ability to use glucose and produce neurotransmitters, such as serotonin, which regulate mood.

Additionally, poor skin health can be a visible cue of metabolic issues. Skin conditions such as acne, dryness, or a general lackluster appearance can be related to nutritional deficiencies or hormonal imbalances linked to metabolic health. Similarly, hair loss or brittle nails can also indicate nutrient absorption issues or a shortage of vital minerals and vitamins necessary for maintaining these tissues. A constant feeling of cold or difficulty in regulating body temperature can indicate thyroid problems, often associated with metabolic rate. The thyroid gland plays a crucial role in metabolism, and its dysfunction can lead to feeling unusually cold or having an intolerance to cold temperatures, a symptom frequently observed in hypothyroidism. Recognizing these signs requires attentiveness to one's body and its signals. It is essential to not dismiss subtle shifts in physical and mental states, as they can provide critical clues about metabolic health. Regular monitoring of these symptoms, combined with laboratory tests to measure blood glucose levels, hormone profiles, and other relevant markers, can provide a comprehensive picture of metabolic function. Addressing suboptimal metabolism involves a multi-faceted approach, emphasizing dietary adjustments, physical activity, stress management, and potentially medical interventions. By adopting a lifestyle that supports optimal metabolic function, individuals can enhance their body's efficiency in using energy, maintaining weight, regulating hormones, and overall health. Awareness and early recognition of the signs of metabolic distress empower individuals to maintain not just metabolic balance but overall health and well-being, paving the way for a healthier and more vibrant life.

Chapter 2: Adopting a Lifestyle that Promotes Optimal Metabolism

Lifestyle and Metabolic Health: What Works and What Doesn't

In the quest for optimal health, understanding the pivotal role of lifestyle in shaping metabolic processes is essential. Metabolic health is not determined solely by genetic predisposition or sporadic efforts toward healthy living; it is the outcome of sustained lifestyle choices that either foster or hinder bodily functions. This section delves into the elements of lifestyle that positively influence metabolic health and highlights common misconceptions and ineffective practices.

The relationship between lifestyle and metabolic health is multifaceted, encompassing diet, physical activity, sleep, stress management, and environmental factors. Each of these components can significantly influence metabolic functions such as glucose regulation, lipid profiles, and hormone levels. For instance, a balanced diet rich in nutrients supports metabolic enzymes and hormone production, while regular physical activity improves insulin sensitivity and boosts metabolic rate.

What Works:

1. **Regular Physical Activity:** Engaging in regular exercise is one of the most effective ways to boost metabolic health. Activities like aerobic exercises, strength training, and flexibility workouts not only burn calories but also improve the body's ability to regulate blood sugar and manage weight. The American Heart Association recommends at least 150 minutes of moderate aerobic activity or 75 minutes of vigorous activity per week, supplemented by muscle-strengthening activities on two or more days.

2. **Balanced, Nutrient-Dense Diet:** Consuming a diet that emphasizes whole foods such as vegetables, fruits, lean proteins, and whole grains is crucial. Such foods provide essential nutrients and fiber, which aid in regulating digestion and maintaining stable blood sugar levels. Moreover, integrating healthy fats from sources like avocados, nuts, and olive oil can support hormone health and cellular function.

3. **Adequate Sleep:** Quality sleep is critical in maintaining metabolic health. During sleep, the body repairs itself and balances key hormones, including those responsible for appetite regulation. Adults should aim for 7-9 hours of sleep per night to support these processes effectively.

4. **Stress Reduction:** Chronic stress can severely disrupt metabolic health, leading to increased cortisol levels and insulin resistance. Practices such as mindfulness, yoga, and adequate leisure can mitigate stress and promote a more balanced metabolic state.

5. **Environmental Considerations:** Reducing exposure to environmental toxins such as pollutants, chemicals in food and water, and excessive noise and light can also

contribute to better metabolic health. These toxins can interfere with hormonal balances and metabolic functions.

What Doesn't Work:

1. **Fad Diets:** While trendy diets promise quick weight loss and health benefits, they often lack scientific support and can result in nutritional imbalances that harm metabolic health. Diets that severely restrict calorie intake or eliminate whole food groups can lead to metabolic slowdown, muscle loss, and can even exacerbate health issues.

2. **Overtraining:** While regular exercise is beneficial, excessive physical activity can lead to overtraining syndrome, which negatively affects metabolism. Symptoms include fatigue, decreased performance, and increased susceptibility to injuries.

3. **Neglecting Mental Health:** Often overlooked in discussions about metabolic health, mental well-being is crucial. Anxiety, depression, and other mental health issues can lead to hormonal imbalances and adverse metabolic effects.

4. **Sleep Debt and Poor Sleep Hygiene:** Sacrificing sleep for extended work hours or social activities can disrupt circadian rhythms and hormonal balances, leading to poor metabolic health.

5. **Ignoring Genetic Predispositions:** While lifestyle is influential, ignoring genetic predispositions related to metabolism can be detrimental. For instance, individuals with a family history of diabetes should pay particular attention to their carbohydrate intake and glycemic load.

Effective lifestyle strategies for improving metabolic health are neither temporary fixes nor one-size-fits-all solutions. They require a comprehensive, tailored approach that considers individual needs and preferences. Incorporating sustainable, scientifically-backed practices into daily life is the best way to enhance metabolic functions and achieve lasting health benefits. This understanding of what genuinely works and what doesn't is fundamental to adopting a lifestyle that promotes optimal metabolism. By making informed choices, individuals can significantly influence their health trajectory, paving the way for a healthier, more vibrant life.

Practical Ways to Modify Lifestyle to Support Metabolism

Adopting a lifestyle that promotes optimal metabolic health involves more than understanding the underlying principles; it requires actionable strategies that can be integrated into daily life. This section outlines practical ways to modify lifestyle habits to support and enhance metabolic function, crucial for maintaining energy, managing weight, and preventing disease.

Establishing a Routine for Physical Activity

Physical activity is paramount for boosting metabolism. It enhances insulin sensitivity, increases muscle mass, and elevates the rate at which your body burns calories, even while at rest. However, the key to sustaining an exercise routine is integration into your daily life:

- **Consistency Over Intensity**: Start with activities you enjoy and can perform regularly. Whether it's walking, cycling, swimming, or group sports, the goal is to stay active consistently rather than pushing through high-intensity workouts sporadically.
- **Incorporate Strength Training**: Muscle tissue burns more calories than fat tissue. Incorporating strength training a few times a week can help build muscle mass and increase resting metabolic rate.
- **Flexibility and Recovery**: Including flexibility exercises like yoga or Pilates helps maintain muscle elasticity and prevent injuries. Recovery days are also vital to allow muscles to repair and grow.

Nutritional Adjustments for Metabolic Support

Diet plays a critical role in metabolic health. What you eat can either fuel your body efficiently or lead to energy crashes and health issues:

- **Eat Balanced Meals**: Structure your meals to include a good balance of proteins, fats, and carbohydrates. This balance helps regulate blood sugar levels and provides a steady energy supply.
- **Focus on Whole Foods**: Minimize intake of processed foods, which often contain unhealthy fats, sugars, and additives that can disrupt metabolic health. Instead, focus on whole foods like vegetables, fruits, whole grains, and lean proteins.
- **Hydrate Wisely**: Staying hydrated is essential for metabolic processes, but the choice of beverages can impact your metabolism. Water is the best choice; avoid sugary drinks and limit caffeine and alcohol, which can interfere with sleep and, subsequently, metabolism.

Optimizing Sleep Patterns

Quality sleep is as vital as diet and exercise for metabolic health. Poor sleep can disrupt hormones that regulate appetite and metabolism:

- **Establish a Sleep Schedule**: Going to bed and waking up at the same time every day helps regulate your body's internal clock and improves your sleep quality.
- **Create a Restful Environment**: Ensure your sleeping environment is conducive to rest. It should be cool, quiet, and dark. Consider using blackout curtains, eye masks, or white noise machines if necessary.
- **Limit Stimulants**: Avoid caffeine and heavy meals close to bedtime as they can disrupt sleep. Also, limit exposure to blue light from screens in the evening.

Managing Stress Effectively

Chronic stress can wreak havoc on your metabolism by raising cortisol levels, which can lead to weight gain and other health issues:

- **Regular Relaxation and Mindfulness Practices**: Engage in activities that reduce stress, such as meditation, deep-breathing exercises, or hobbies that you enjoy.
- **Physical Activity**: Exercise is also a powerful stress reliever. Even short bouts of activity can release endorphins, improving mood and reducing stress.
- **Connect Socially**: Maintaining social connections can provide emotional support and reduce stress. Regular interaction with friends, family, or community groups can be beneficial.

Environmental and Lifestyle Considerations

The environment you live in can also impact your metabolic health:

- **Minimize Toxin Exposure**: Be aware of toxins in your environment, such as air and water pollutants and chemical cleaners, which can affect your metabolic health. Opt for natural cleaning products and ensure proper ventilation in your living spaces.
- **Mindful Technology Use**: Prolonged sedentary behavior, often associated with excessive screen time, can negatively impact metabolic health. Be mindful of the time spent inactive, and make a conscious effort to move regularly throughout the day.

Incorporating these practical strategies into daily routines can lead to significant improvements in metabolic health. It's about making small, sustainable changes that enhance your body's natural processes, leading to lasting health benefits. By modifying your lifestyle to support your metabolism, you're not just improving your physical health but also enhancing your overall quality of life.

Principles of Metabolic Nutrition

Metabolic nutrition forms the bedrock of a lifestyle that promotes optimal metabolism, focusing on dietary patterns that fuel the body efficiently while supporting overall health. This approach goes beyond simple calorie counting to consider how foods affect various metabolic processes, including energy production, hormonal balance, and enzymatic reactions. By understanding and applying the principles of metabolic nutrition, individuals can tailor their diets to enhance their metabolic health, leading to increased energy, improved weight management, and a reduced risk of chronic diseases.

The first principle of metabolic nutrition is the balance of macronutrients–carbohydrates, proteins, and fats. Each macronutrient plays a unique role in metabolism:

- **Carbohydrates** are the body's primary energy source. They break down into glucose, which fuels brain function and physical activity. However, not all carbohydrates are created equal. Complex carbohydrates, such as those found in whole grains, vegetables, and legumes, release glucose gradually, helping to maintain steady blood sugar levels and prevent insulin spikes.
- **Proteins** are crucial for building and repairing tissues and are involved in producing hormones and enzymes that regulate metabolic processes. Including a protein source at each meal can help stabilize blood sugar levels and sustain satiety, reducing the likelihood of overeating.

- **Fats** are essential for absorbing fat-soluble vitamins and providing energy. Healthy fats, such as those from avocados, nuts, seeds, and oily fish, also play a role in reducing inflammation, which is linked to metabolic disorders such as type 2 diabetes and obesity.

The second principle is dietary diversity. Consuming a wide variety of foods ensures an adequate intake of all necessary nutrients, which supports metabolic health. Diversity in the diet aids not just in nutrient absorption but also in maintaining a healthy gut microbiome, which research has shown to be crucial for metabolic function and overall health. The third principle involves the timing of meals, which can significantly influence metabolic processes. Eating regular meals helps to maintain blood sugar levels, while erratic eating patterns can disrupt metabolic balance. Recent studies suggest that aligning meal times with circadian rhythms, such as eating larger meals earlier in the day, may improve metabolic health by syncing meal times with the body's natural hormonal fluctuations. Hydration is another critical component of metabolic nutrition. Water is essential for numerous metabolic functions, including digestion and the transportation of nutrients. Maintaining proper hydration helps optimize these processes and enhances cellular function.

Another principle is the reduction of sugar and processed foods. High intake of added sugars has been linked to various metabolic issues, including poor insulin response, higher body fat, and elevated triglyceride levels. Processed foods often contain unhealthy fats and additives that can disrupt metabolic health. Reducing these in your diet and focusing on fresh, whole foods can significantly improve metabolic responses.

Metabolic nutrition also emphasizes the importance of micronutrients—vitamins and minerals that catalyze many chemical reactions in the body. For example, magnesium plays a role in over 300 enzymatic reactions, including those that regulate blood sugar and blood pressure levels. Similarly, B vitamins are crucial for energy metabolism, and their adequate intake supports cellular energy production. Implementing these principles requires mindfulness and commitment. It involves making informed choices about what to eat, when to eat, and how much to eat. It also means being aware of the body's cues. Over time, these choices become part of a sustainable lifestyle, not just a temporary diet.

In conclusion, metabolic nutrition isn't about restrictive eating or following fleeting diet trends. Instead, it's about understanding how different foods and eating patterns affect your body's metabolic processes. By embracing these principles, individuals can enhance their body's natural metabolic functions, which leads to better health outcomes and a more vibrant, energetic life. This comprehensive approach to diet provides the tools necessary to make informed, health-promoting dietary choices that support lifelong metabolic health.

Foods to Favor and Foods to Avoid

In the pursuit of optimal metabolic health, understanding which foods to incorporate into your diet and which to limit is crucial. This guidance is not just about reducing calorie intake but about making strategic choices that enhance metabolic functions and contribute to overall well-being. The focus here is on selecting foods that nurture the body, promote energy balance, and support long-term health.

Foods to Favor

Whole Grains: Unlike their refined counterparts, whole grains retain all parts of the seed-the bran, germ, and endosperm. Foods like brown rice, quinoa, oats, and whole wheat provide essential nutrients such as fiber, vitamins, and minerals that help regulate blood sugar and improve insulin sensitivity.

Lean Proteins: Incorporating lean sources of protein such as chicken, turkey, fish, legumes, and tofu can boost satiety and help in maintaining muscle mass, which is vital for a healthy metabolism. Fish such as salmon and mackerel also provide omega-3 fatty acids, which are known for their anti-inflammatory properties.

Healthy Fats: Fats are crucial for brain health and energy, but the type of fat matters. Monounsaturated and polyunsaturated fats, found in avocados, nuts, seeds, and olive oil, promote heart health and support insulin sensitivity. These fats are not only essential for nutrient absorption but also help stabilize energy levels throughout the day.

Fruits and Vegetables: Rich in fiber, vitamins, minerals, and antioxidants, fruits and vegetables are fundamental for an anti-inflammatory diet. They provide the necessary compounds that help combat oxidative stress-an underlying factor in metabolic disorders such as obesity and type 2 diabetes.

Fermented Foods: Foods like yogurt, kefir, sauerkraut, and kimchi are rich in probiotics, which are beneficial for gut health. A healthy gut microbiome is essential for proper digestion and can significantly impact metabolic health and immunity.

Foods to Avoid

Sugary Foods and Beverages: High intake of sugar, especially added sugars found in sodas, candies, and baked goods, can lead to spikes in blood sugar and insulin levels, contributing to weight gain and insulin resistance. These foods offer little nutritional benefit and are often high in calories, which can disrupt metabolic health.

Refined Carbohydrates: Foods such as white bread, pastries, and other products made from refined grains are stripped of their fiber and nutrients during processing. They are quickly digested, leading to rapid increases in blood sugar and insulin levels, which can strain metabolic processes over time.

Trans Fats: Often found in fried foods, baked goods, and processed snack foods, trans fats are linked to increased risk of heart disease and inflammation. These fats can alter cell membrane structure and function, which negatively affects metabolism.

Alcohol: While moderate alcohol consumption might have some health benefits, excessive intake can be harmful. Alcohol can interfere with liver function and fat metabolism. It also adds extra calories to the diet, which can lead to weight gain and disrupt normal metabolic processes.

High-Sodium Processed Foods: Excessive sodium consumption, often found in processed foods, can lead to high blood pressure and increase the risk of cardiovascular disease. These foods also tend to be high in unhealthy fats and calories, which can impede metabolic health.

The distinction between foods to favor and foods to avoid is not about restrictive dieting but about making informed, mindful choices that enhance metabolic efficiency. By focusing on nutrient-dense foods and limiting those that offer little nutritional value, individuals can manage their metabolic health more effectively. This approach not only supports metabolic processes but also aligns with a holistic view of health that embraces a variety of foods and flavors to nourish the body and enrich the dining experience. Adopting these dietary practices is a step towards sustained health and vitality, providing the body with the essential nutrients it needs to function optimally while avoiding those that hinder its performance.

The Role of Macronutrients

Understanding the role of macronutrients—carbohydrates, proteins, and fats—is fundamental to adopting a lifestyle that promotes optimal metabolism. These nutrients are the cornerstone of nutritional science and are essential for the body's energy production, growth, and cellular functions. Each macronutrient plays a specific role in metabolic health, influencing everything from energy levels and body composition to hormonal balance and chronic disease risk.

Carbohydrates

Carbohydrates are often labeled as the primary energy source for the body, especially for the brain and central nervous system. They break down into glucose, which is used immediately for energy or stored in the liver and muscles as glycogen for later use. The quality and type of carbohydrates consumed can significantly impact metabolic health.

Complex Carbohydrates: These are found in foods such as whole grains, legumes, and vegetables. They are rich in fiber, which slows down digestion and provides a steady release of glucose into the bloodstream, leading to more stable blood sugar levels and sustained energy. Fiber also aids in digestive health and has been shown to reduce the risk of chronic diseases such as type 2 diabetes and cardiovascular disease.

Simple Carbohydrates: These include sugars found naturally in fruits and milk, as well as those added during processing. While natural sugars are accompanied by vitamins, minerals, and fiber, added sugars are devoid of these nutrients and can lead to quick spikes in blood glucose levels, contributing to energy crashes and, over time, to insulin resistance.

Proteins

Proteins are vital for more than just muscle repair and growth. They are crucial for the creation of enzymes, hormones, neurotransmitters, and other molecules essential for life. Proteins consist of amino acids, some of which are essential and must be obtained through diet.

Amino Acids: The building blocks of proteins, amino acids play critical roles in nearly every metabolic process in the body. They are necessary for the synthesis of hormones and neurotransmitters that regulate metabolism, mood, and cognitive functions.

Protein Quality: High-quality proteins contain all essential amino acids in sufficient amounts. Animal-based proteins generally provide complete protein, while most plant-based protein sources need to be combined to achieve completeness.

Fats

Fats have been misunderstood, often vilified in the diet culture; however, they are indispensable for health. Fats provide a concentrated source of energy, are essential for the absorption of fat-soluble vitamins, and are necessary for the construction of cell membranes.

Saturated and Unsaturated Fats: Understanding the difference between these can significantly impact health. Saturated fats, found in foods like butter, cheese, and red meat, should be consumed in moderation. Unsaturated fats, which include monounsaturated and polyunsaturated fats, are found in foods like fish, nuts, seeds, and plant oils, and contribute to heart health and reduce inflammation.

Omega-3 Fatty Acids: These are a type of polyunsaturated fat found in fatty fish and flaxseeds, known for their role in decreasing inflammation, lowering heart disease risk, and supporting brain health.

Balancing Macronutrients

The balance of macronutrients can influence metabolic rate, body composition, and overall health. Diets too high in certain macronutrients or lacking in others can lead to metabolic imbalances, weight gain, and increased risk of diseases.

Personalized Nutrition: There is no one-size-fits-all macronutrient ratio that works for everyone. Individual needs can vary based on age, gender, activity level, and health goals. A balanced diet that includes an appropriate mix of all macronutrients tailored to individual preferences and needs is crucial for maintaining optimal metabolic health.

Metabolic Flexibility: This refers to the body's ability to switch between using carbohydrates or fats as the primary energy source efficiently. Enhancing metabolic flexibility can improve overall energy utilization and metabolic health.

In summary, carbohydrates, proteins, and fats each play distinct and vital roles in supporting metabolic health. By understanding and managing the intake of these macronutrients, individuals can optimize their metabolism, enhance their health, and improve their quality of life. The strategic integration of these macronutrients into the diet not only supports immediate metabolic needs but also lays the groundwork for long-term health and vitality.

Chapter 3: The Diet for Optimal Metabolism

Basics of a Diet that Supports Metabolism

When we think about a diet that bolsters our metabolic health, it's essential to recognize that this isn't merely about eating less or more; it's about eating right. The foundation of such a diet hinges on understanding how foods interact with our body's natural processes to either fuel or impede its functionality.

The human body is akin to a complex biochemical laboratory, constantly processing nutrients, hormones, and enzymes in a fine-tuned balance that supports life's various functions. Metabolism, at its core, refers to how our bodies convert food into the energy it needs to function and then how it manages the waste products from this process. Therefore, a diet that supports metabolism effectively encourages optimal energy use and minimal waste. Key to this approach is focusing on foods that our bodies can use efficiently. These foods often share common characteristics: they are nutrient-dense, naturally low in sugars, high in fiber, and full of the vitamins and minerals that aid metabolic pathways. Consuming a variety of such foods ensures that the body receives a broad spectrum of nutrients essential for its complex systems. One critical element in a metabolism-supporting diet is the balance of macronutrients—carbohydrates, fats, and proteins. Each plays a unique role in energy production and must be consumed in ratios that reflect your personal health needs and activity levels. Carbohydrates, for instance, are the body's primary energy source. However, not all carbs are created equal. Complex carbohydrates, such as those found in whole grains, legumes, and vegetables, break down slowly in the body, providing a steady stream of energy and keeping blood sugar levels stable. Fats are often vilified, but they are essential to health as they support cellular function and provide a concentrated energy source. The key is to choose healthy fats, such as those from avocados, nuts, seeds, and fish. These fats not only support metabolism but also help with the absorption of essential vitamins. Proteins are the building blocks of muscle and are crucial for repair and growth. They also play a significant role in metabolic health as they can influence satiety and are involved in the production of enzymes and hormones. Including a moderate amount of protein from diverse sources can help maintain muscle mass and support metabolic processes.

Another pillar of a metabolism-supporting diet is hydration. Water is essential for all forms of life and plays a myriad of roles in our bodies, including aiding digestion and nutrient absorption, regulating body temperature, and detoxifying cells. It's crucial to drink adequate amounts of water throughout the day to support these functions. Beyond the types of food, the timing of meals can also impact metabolic health. Regular, spaced-out meals and snacks help maintain blood sugar levels and prevent the peaks and troughs that can lead to metabolic slowdown. Intermittent fasting, where eating is restricted to certain hours of the day, has also shown promise in improving metabolic outcomes by aligning food intake with natural circadian rhythms, thereby optimizing the times when the body is best prepared to process nutrients. Understanding the impact of each food type and nutrient timing can be empowering. It allows individuals to make informed choices that align with their body's needs. However, the journey to optimizing metabolism through diet is highly individual. What works for one person may not work for another due to variations in genetics, lifestyle, age, and health status. Thus, to construct a diet that genuinely supports your metabolic health, it is advisable to experiment with these principles under the guidance of healthcare professionals. They can help tailor a nutritional plan that not only considers your metabolic needs but also fits your lifestyle and food preferences.

By embracing a diet rich in a variety of nutrient-dense foods, balanced in macronutrients, and aligned with your body's natural rhythms, you can enhance your metabolism, thereby promoting greater energy levels, better health, and an improved quality of life. This holistic approach does not just change what you eat, it transforms how you live, leading to a more vibrant, healthful existence.

Managing Blood Sugar Spikes

Managing blood sugar levels is a critical aspect of any dietary strategy aimed at enhancing metabolic health. Fluctuations in blood sugar can lead to swings in energy levels, mood disturbances, and over time, can strain the body's metabolic processes, potentially leading to insulin resistance and diabetes. Understanding how to manage these spikes through dietary choices is not just about avoiding sugar but about creating a balanced approach to eating that stabilizes blood sugar levels throughout the day. Blood sugar control is fundamental because it affects how we feel and perform on a daily basis. When blood sugar levels spike, the body responds by secreting insulin to help transport glucose into cells. However, frequent high spikes followed by sharp drops can lead to the cells becoming less responsive to insulin. This condition, known as insulin resistance, is a precursor to more serious metabolic issues, including type 2 diabetes and cardiovascular diseases. To manage blood sugar effectively, it's essential to focus on the glycemic impact of foods. The glycemic index (GI) is a valuable tool in this regard, rating foods on how quickly they raise blood sugar levels after eating. Foods with a high GI score cause rapid spikes, whereas those with a low GI provide a slower release of energy. Integrating more low-GI foods into your diet, such as whole grains, legumes, and most vegetables, helps maintain steady blood sugar levels.

Fiber plays a crucial role in this context. Dietary fiber, particularly soluble fiber, can slow the absorption of sugar, helping to improve blood sugar levels and lower insulin spikes. Foods rich in high-quality fiber–such as oats, beans, lentils, berries, and apples–not only extend digestion times but also contribute to a feeling of fullness, which can help control overall food intake. Incorporating healthy fats and proteins in meals can also temper blood sugar elevations. Both macronutrients have minimal direct impact on blood glucose levels and can help slow the digestion of carbohydrates. For example, adding a source of healthy fats like avocado or a handful of nuts to a meal, or including a moderate portion of protein like chicken or fish, can reduce the overall glycemic load of a meal. Meal composition and timing are equally significant. Eating balanced meals at regular intervals during the day can prevent the peaks and valleys that lead to metabolic distress. Skipping meals, on the other hand, often leads to overeating later, which can cause a significant surge in blood sugar. Regular, balanced meals help maintain a steady energy intake and metabolism, which supports overall metabolic health. Furthermore, the size of the meal and its composition are important. Large meals can cause significant blood sugar fluctuations, so it might be more beneficial to eat smaller, more frequent meals. This strategy can help stabilize blood sugar levels throughout the day and is especially beneficial for individuals who are managing insulin resistance or diabetes. Another factor is the physical state of the food consumed. Whole foods, as opposed to processed ones, generally have a lower glycemic index and contain more nutrients and fiber. Processing can strip away beneficial components like fiber and add elements like sugar, which can significantly affect a food's impact on blood sugar levels. Beverages also play a role in managing blood sugar. Sugary drinks, including sodas and fruit juices, can cause immediate and dramatic increases in blood sugar. Replacing these with water, herbal teas, or seltzers can drastically reduce sugar intake and help in managing blood sugar spikes. In the context of dietary management, monitoring your body's response to different foods can be incredibly insightful. Everyone's body reacts differently to certain foods; what may cause a spike in one person could have a minimal effect on another. Keeping a food diary and noting how you feel after eating specific foods can help identify patterns and guide more personalized dietary choices. Lastly, lifestyle factors such as physical activity and stress management should not be underestimated in their ability to influence blood sugar levels. Regular physical activity helps increase insulin sensitivity, meaning the body needs less insulin to manage blood sugar levels. Meanwhile, stress prompts the release of hormones such as cortisol, which can increase blood sugar levels.

By understanding and managing these factors, you can effectively stabilize blood sugar levels, leading to improved energy levels, better mood stability, and a robust metabolic profile. This proactive approach to diet and lifestyle not only supports metabolic health but also enhances overall quality of life, promoting long-term well-being and vitality.

How to Personalize Your Diet Based on Individual Needs

Personalizing a diet to meet individual health needs is a complex yet rewarding approach that integrates one's unique physiological, lifestyle, and personal preferences to create a sustainable eating plan. This tailored approach not only optimizes metabolic health but also enhances the overall well-being of an individual. Every person is unique—not just in their DNA, but also in their daily energy demands, health history, environmental interactions, and even taste preferences. A diet that works wonders for one might not be effective for another. This realization has given rise to the concept of personalized nutrition, a strategy that assesses and utilizes various health markers to recommend dietary choices that best support individual metabolic needs.

The first step in personalizing your diet is to understand the specific factors that influence your health and metabolism. These can include age, gender, genetic predisposition, current health status, activity level, and even microbiome composition. For instance, a young athlete may require a higher proportion of carbohydrates for energy, while someone with a sedentary lifestyle might need to focus more on proteins and fibers to enhance satiety and manage weight. Genetic testing can offer profound insights into how your body processes certain foods and can guide dietary adjustments that cater to your metabolic health. For example, if you have a genetic variation that affects how you metabolize caffeine, you might need to adjust your coffee consumption accordingly to avoid sleep disturbances and potential increases in blood pressure. Moreover, understanding any existing health conditions is crucial for personalizing your diet. Conditions such as diabetes, heart disease, or thyroid imbalances can significantly influence your dietary needs. In such cases, the diet must be tailored not only to manage symptoms but also to prevent disease progression.

Another key element in personalizing your diet is recognizing and respecting your body's hunger and satiety signals. Learning to listen to your body's cues can help regulate food intake naturally without overeating or restricting. This requires a mindful approach to eating, where the focus is on the quality of the diet, recognizing hunger levels, and understanding emotional eating triggers. Personalization also extends to accommodating lifestyle factors such as work schedules, family life, and even social commitments, which can influence meal timing and choices. For instance, someone who works night shifts may need a different eating schedule and type of diet to maintain their health compared to someone with a standard day job. In addition to these physiological and lifestyle considerations, dietary preferences and intolerances must also be taken into account. This includes not only taste preferences but also ethical beliefs and food allergies or intolerances. Creating a diet plan that respects these aspects while ensuring nutritional adequacy is essential for long-term adherence and satisfaction. To effectively personalize your diet, it may be beneficial to work with a dietitian or a nutritionist who can help interpret complex health information and translate it into a practical and personalized eating plan. They can also help monitor your health indicators, adjust your diet as needed, and provide guidance on meal planning and preparation.

Moreover, the use of technology in tracking and analyzing dietary intake and health outcomes can enhance the personalization process. Various apps and devices allow for the monitoring of meals, physical activity, sleep patterns, and even blood sugar levels, offering a comprehensive view of how different aspects of lifestyle and diet interact with one another. It's also important to revisit and adjust the diet plan periodically as your health needs, lifestyle, and preferences change. This iterative process ensures that the diet remains aligned with your evolving health goals and circumstances. In sum, personalizing your diet is about creating a dynamic eating plan that responds to your unique health requirements, preferences, and lifestyle. By focusing on individual needs rather than conforming to one-size-fits-all dietary guidelines, you can optimize your metabolic health and enhance your overall quality of life. This approach empowers individuals to make informed and conscious food choices that support both their immediate and long-term health objectives.

Long-term Benefits of Targeted Nutrition

Targeted nutrition is a strategic approach that aligns dietary intake with specific health goals to optimize metabolism and enhance overall well-being. This concept goes beyond basic nutritional needs, focusing on the long-term benefits that come from a diet specifically tailored to support metabolic processes, disease prevention, and an enriched quality of life. By understanding and implementing targeted nutrition, individuals can experience profound changes that not only improve their current health status but also protect against future health issues.

One of the most compelling benefits of targeted nutrition is its impact on metabolic health. A diet that is carefully designed to meet individual metabolic needs can improve the efficiency of metabolic processes such as energy production, fat burning, and blood sugar regulation. Over time, this leads to more balanced energy levels throughout the day, reduced feelings of fatigue, and a lower risk of metabolic syndromes such as diabetes and obesity. This is because when the diet is aligned with one's metabolic profile, the body can more efficiently process and utilize nutrients, preventing excessive fat storage and stabilizing blood glucose levels. Moreover, targeted nutrition plays a crucial role in preventing chronic diseases. By focusing on nutrients that support heart health, such as omega-3 fatty acids, antioxidants, and soluble fiber, individuals can significantly reduce their risk of cardiovascular diseases. Diets rich in these nutrients have been shown to lower blood pressure, reduce cholesterol levels, and improve arterial health, all of which contribute to a healthier heart and circulatory system.

The benefits of targeted nutrition also extend to mental health. Nutrients such as omega-3 fatty acids, B vitamins, and amino acids play essential roles in brain function and can influence mood, cognitive function, and overall mental health. For instance, studies have shown that omega-3 fatty acids help reduce symptoms of depression and anxiety, while B vitamins are crucial for energy production and maintaining proper nerve function. By ensuring that the diet includes these vital nutrients, individuals can maintain optimal brain health and improve their psychological well-being. Targeted nutrition is also integral to maintaining a healthy immune system. A diet that includes a wide range of vitamins, minerals, and antioxidants boosts the body's natural defenses against infectious diseases. Vitamins such as Vitamin C and Vitamin D, along with minerals like zinc and selenium, are known for their immune-enhancing properties. Regular intake of these nutrients can fortify the immune system, reduce the incidence of illness, and ensure faster recovery when sick. Additionally, the anti-aging effects of targeted nutrition cannot be overlooked. Nutrients that combat oxidative stress and inflammation, such as antioxidants found in berries and leafy greens, help protect the body's cells from damage. This cellular protection is vital for reducing the risk of age-related diseases such as Alzheimer's, arthritis, and age-related vision loss. Moreover, a diet rich in antioxidants can contribute to healthier skin, reduced wrinkles, and a more youthful appearance, reflecting how targeted nutrition can influence physical signs of aging. Another significant benefit of targeted nutrition is its role in enhancing physical performance and recovery. For athletes or physically active individuals, a diet that includes optimal amounts of proteins, carbohydrates, and electrolytes can enhance performance, promote muscle recovery, and reduce fatigue. By aligning nutritional intake with physical demands, individuals can maximize their athletic performance and decrease the risk of injury. Finally, targeted nutrition supports reproductive health. Nutrients such as folic acid, iron, and calcium are essential for a healthy pregnancy and can influence fetal development and maternal health. By ensuring adequate intake of these and other critical nutrients, prospective mothers can enhance their chances of a healthy pregnancy and childbirth. In conclusion, the long-term benefits of targeted nutrition are extensive and impactful. By tailoring dietary choices to meet specific health and metabolic needs, individuals can enhance their metabolic efficiency, prevent chronic diseases, support mental and immune health, slow aging, boost physical performance, and improve reproductive health. This holistic approach to nutrition not only improves the quality of life in the present but also sets a foundation for sustained health and vitality in the years to come.

RECIPES

Energizing Breakfasts

Coffee Chia Pudding with Coconut and Pecans

Preparation Time: 15 minutes, **Chill Time:** 4 hours, **Servings:** 2

Ingredients:

- 1/4 cup chia seeds (Salvia hispanica)
- 1 cup unsweetened coconut milk (Cocos nucifera)
- 1/2 cup brewed coffee, cooled (Coffea arabica)
- 2 tbsp. crushed pecans (Carya illinoinensis)
- 1 tbsp. unsweetened shredded coconut (Cocos nucifera)
- 1/4 tsp. vanilla extract (Vanilla planifolia)
- Sweetener of choice (e.g., stevia or erythritol), to taste

Nutritional Values:

Nutrient	Per Serving
Calories	215 kcal
Protein	4 g
Carbohydrates	12 g
Fats	16 g
Dietary Fiber	8 g

Procedure:

1. In a medium bowl, combine chia seeds, coconut milk, and brewed coffee. Mix thoroughly to prevent clumping.
2. Stir in vanilla extract and sweetener to taste.
3. Divide the mixture into two serving dishes. Refrigerate for at least 4 hours, or until the pudding achieves a gel-like consistency.
4. Prior to serving, top each pudding with crushed pecans and shredded coconut for added texture and flavor.

Tips:

- For a stronger coffee flavor, increase the amount of brewed coffee to 3/4 cup and reduce the coconut milk by a corresponding amount.
- This pudding can be prepared in advance and stored in the refrigerator for up to 5 days, making it a convenient option for quick breakfasts or snacks.

Green Shakshuka with Spinach and Avocado

Preparation Time: 20 minutes, **Cooking Time:** 15 minutes, **Servings:** 4

Ingredients:

- 1 small onion, finely chopped
- 2 cloves garlic, minced
- 2 cups fresh spinach, roughly chopped
- 1 medium zucchini, diced
- 1/2 tsp ground cumin
- 1/2 tsp coriander
- 4 large eggs
- 1 ripe avocado, sliced
- Salt and pepper, to taste
- Fresh herbs for garnish

Nutritional Values:

Nutrient	Per Serving
Calories	180 kcal
Protein	8 g
Carbohydrates	10 g
Fats	12 g
Dietary Fiber	5 g

Procedure:

1. Heat the olive oil in a large skillet over medium heat. Add the chopped onion and sauté until translucent, about 5 minutes.

2. Add the minced garlic, zucchini, and spices. Cook for another 5 minutes until the zucchini begins to soften.

3. Stir in the chopped spinach and cook until it wilts, about 3 minutes.

4. Create four wells in the vegetable mixture and crack an egg into each well. Season with salt and pepper.

5. Cover the skillet and cook on low heat for about 5-7 minutes, or until the eggs are cooked to your liking.

6. Remove from heat, top with sliced avocado and fresh herbs before serving.

Tips:

- Add a splash of water to the skillet before covering to help steam the eggs to perfection.
- For a dairy-free creamy texture, blend part of the avocado into the vegetable mix before adding the eggs.

Almond Flour Pancakes with Sugar-Free Blueberry Syrup

Preparation Time: 10 minutes, **Cooking Time:** 15 minutes, **Servings:** 4

Ingredients:

- 1 cup almond flour
- 2 large eggs
- 1/4 cup unsweetened almond milk
- 1 tsp baking powder
- 1/4 tsp salt
- 1 tbsp erythritol (or another sugar substitute)
- 1/2 tsp vanilla extract
- Non-stick cooking spray or butter for greasing
- **For the syrup:**
    - 1 cup fresh or frozen blueberries
    - 1/4 cup water
    - 2 tbsp erythritol
- 1/2 tsp lemon juice

Nutritional Values:

Nutrient	Per Serving
Calories	235 kcal
Protein	9 g
Carbohydrates	12 g
Fats	18 g
Dietary Fiber	4 g

Procedure:

1. In a mixing bowl, whisk together almond flour, baking powder, salt, erythritol, and vanilla extract. Beat in eggs and almond milk until the batter is smooth.

2. Heat a non-stick skillet over medium heat and lightly grease with cooking spray or butter.

3. Pour 1/4 cup of batter for each pancake onto the skillet. Cook for about 2-3 minutes per side or until golden brown and cooked through.

4. For the syrup, combine blueberries, water, erythritol, and lemon juice in a small saucepan over medium heat. Bring to a simmer and cook until the berries break down and the syrup thickens, about 10 minutes.

5. Serve pancakes hot with warm blueberry syrup.

Tips:

- If the pancake batter is too thick, adjust by adding a little more almond milk until the desired consistency is reached. To keep pancakes warm while making the entire batch, preheat your oven to 200°F (about 93°C) and place cooked pancakes on a baking sheet in the oven.

Avocado Toast with Smoked Salmon and Radishes

Preparation Time: 10 minutes, **Servings:** 2

Ingredients:

- 2 slices of whole grain bread
- 1 ripe avocado, peeled and pitted
- 4 oz smoked salmon
- 4-6 radishes, thinly sliced
- 1 tbsp capers
- 1/2 small red onion, thinly sliced
- Fresh dill, chopped
- Lemon wedges for serving
- Salt and pepper to taste

- **Nutritional Values:**

Nutrient	Per Serving
Calories	320 kcal
Protein	15 g
Carbohydrates	30 g
Fats	17 g
Dietary Fiber	9 g

Procedure:

1. Toast the whole grain bread slices until golden and crispy.
2. In a small bowl, mash the avocado with a fork until creamy. Season with salt and pepper to taste.
3. Spread the mashed avocado evenly over each slice of toast.
4. Arrange the smoked salmon over the avocado. Top with sliced radishes, red onion, and capers.
5. Garnish with fresh dill and serve with lemon wedges on the side.

Tips:

- For an added kick, drizzle a little lemon juice over the avocado before adding the toppings.
- Opt for high-quality, sustainably sourced smoked salmon to ensure the best flavor and environmental consideration.

Baked Eggs with Kale and Turkey Sausage

Preparation Time: 10 minutes, **Cooking Time:** 20 minutes, **Servings:** 4

Ingredients:

- 1 tbsp olive oil
- 4 turkey sausage links, casing removed and crumbled
- 2 cups kale, chopped
- 1 clove garlic, minced
- 4 large eggs
- 1/4 cup grated Parmesan cheese
- Salt and pepper to taste
- Crushed red pepper flakes (optional)

Nutritional Values:

Nutrient	Per Serving
Calories	300 kcal
Protein	22 g
Carbohydrates	8 g
Fats	20 g
Dietary Fiber	2 g

Procedure:

1. Preheat oven to 400°F (200°C).
2. Heat olive oil in a large oven-safe skillet over medium heat. Add the crumbled turkey sausage and cook until browned, about 5 minutes.
3. Add the chopped kale and minced garlic to the skillet. Cook until the kale is wilted and the garlic is fragrant, about 3 minutes.
4. Create four wells in the mixture and crack an egg into each well. Sprinkle Parmesan cheese, salt, and pepper over the top.
5. Transfer the skillet to the oven and bake for 10-12 minutes, or until the egg whites are set but the yolks are still runny.
6. Remove from the oven and sprinkle with red pepper flakes if using.

Tips:

- Ensure that the skillet is hot before adding the eggs, as this helps to cook the eggs evenly and prevent sticking.
- Adjust the baking time if you prefer your yolks more or less set.

Pumpkin Pancakes with Coconut Syrup and Cinnamon

Preparation Time: 15 minutes, **Cooking Time:** 10 minutes, **Servings:** 4

Ingredients:

- 1 cup all-purpose flour
- 1/2 cup pumpkin puree
- 1 1/4 cups milk
- 1 large egg
- 2 tbsp sugar
- 2 tsp baking powder
- 1/2 tsp cinnamon
- 1/4 tsp nutmeg
- 1/4 tsp salt
- **For the coconut syrup:**
    - 1/2 cup coconut milk
    - 1/4 cup sugar
    - 1/2 tsp vanilla extract

Nutritional Values:

Nutrient	Per Serving
Calories	280 kcal
Protein	6 g
Carbohydrates	40 g
Fats	11 g
Dietary Fiber	2 g

Procedure:

11. In a large mixing bowl, combine flour, sugar, baking powder, cinnamon, nutmeg, and salt.
12. In another bowl, whisk together the pumpkin puree, milk, egg.
13. Pour the wet ingredients into the dry ingredients and stir until just combined; be careful not to overmix.
14. Heat a non-stick skillet over medium heat and lightly grease it with cooking spray or a little oil.
15. Pour 1/4 cup of batter for each pancake onto the skillet. Cook for about 2-3 minutes on each side or until golden brown and the edges are set.
16. For the coconut syrup, combine coconut milk, sugar, and vanilla extract in a small saucepan. Heat over medium heat, stirring frequently, until the sugar is dissolved and the mixture is hot.
17. Serve the pancakes warm, drizzled with the coconut syrup.

- **Tips:**
    - If the pancake batter is too thick, add a bit more milk to reach the desired consistency.
    - You can add a few drops of coconut extract to the pancake batter for a stronger coconut flavor.

Mango Smoothie Bowl with Chia Seeds and Macadamia Nuts

Preparation Time: 10 minutes, **Servings:** 2

Ingredients:

- 2 cups frozen mango chunks
- 1 banana
- 1/2 cup plain Greek yogurt
- 1/2 cup coconut water
- 2 tbsp chia seeds
- 1/4 cup macadamia nuts, chopped
- Optional toppings: sliced kiwi, coconut flakes, honey

- Nutritional Values:

Nutrient	Per Serving
Calories	350 kcal
Protein	8 g
Carbohydrates	53 g
Fats	14 g
Dietary Fiber	7 g

Procedure:

1. In a blender, combine frozen mango chunks, banana, Greek yogurt, and coconut water. Blend until smooth and creamy.

2. Pour the smoothie mixture into two bowls.

3. Sprinkle each bowl evenly with chia seeds and chopped macadamia nuts.

4. Add optional toppings such as sliced kiwi, coconut flakes, or a drizzle of honey if desired.

Tips:

- For a thicker smoothie bowl, use less coconut water or add a scoop of protein powder for additional thickness and protein.
- Freeze the banana beforehand for an extra creamy texture.

Almond Flour Muffins with Blueberries and Lemon Zest

Preparation Time: 15 minutes, **Cooking Time:** 25 minutes, **Servings:** 12 muffins

Ingredients:

- 2 cups almond flour
- 1 tsp baking powder
- 1/4 tsp salt
- 3 large eggs
- 1/3 cup unsweetened almond milk
- 1/4 cup vegetable oil
- 1/2 cup erythritol (or another sugar substitute)
- 1 tsp vanilla extract
- Zest of 1 lemon
- 1 cup blueberries (fresh or frozen)

- **Nutritional Values:**

Nutrient	Per Muffin
Calories	180 kcal
Protein	6 g
Carbohydrates	10 g
Fats	14 g
Dietary Fiber	3 g

Procedure:

1. Preheat oven to 350°F (175°C). Line a muffin tin with paper liners or lightly grease with cooking spray.
2. In a large bowl, whisk together almond flour, baking powder, and salt.
3. In another bowl, beat the eggs with almond milk, vegetable oil, erythritol, vanilla extract, and lemon zest until smooth.
4. Combine the wet ingredients with the dry ingredients and stir until just mixed.
5. Gently fold in the blueberries.
6. Distribute the batter evenly among the prepared muffin cups, filling each about two-thirds full.
7. Bake for 25 minutes, or until the tops are golden and a toothpick inserted into the center of a muffin comes out clean.
8. Allow to cool in the pan for 5 minutes, then transfer to a wire rack to cool completely.

Tips:

- Be careful not to overmix the batter to keep the muffins light and fluffy.
- If using frozen blueberries, do not thaw them before adding to the batter to prevent bleeding.

Asparagus and Prosciutto Egg Casserole

Preparation Time: 15 minutes, **Cooking Time:** 35 minutes, **Servings:** 6

Ingredients:

- 1 tbsp olive oil
- 1 lb asparagus, trimmed and cut into 1-inch pieces
- 6 large eggs
- 1/2 cup full-fat coconut milk
- 6 slices prosciutto, chopped
- 1/2 cup grated Parmesan cheese
- Salt and pepper to taste
- Optional: 1/4 tsp garlic powder or fresh minced garlic

- **Nutritional Values:**

Nutrient	Per Serving
Calories	220 kcal
Protein	15 g
Carbohydrates	4 g
Fats	16 g
Dietary Fiber	1 g

Procedure:

1. Preheat the oven to 375°F (190°C). Grease a medium-sized baking dish with a bit of olive oil.

2. Heat olive oil in a skillet over medium heat. Add the asparagus and cook until tender but still crisp, about 5-7 minutes. If using garlic, add it during the last 2 minutes of cooking.

3. In a large bowl, whisk together eggs, coconut milk, salt, and pepper. Stir in the cooked asparagus, chopped prosciutto, and half of the Parmesan cheese.

4. Pour the mixture into the prepared baking dish and sprinkle with the remaining Parmesan cheese.

5. Bake in the preheated oven for about 25-30 minutes, or until the eggs are set and the top is lightly golden.

6. Let the casserole sit for a few minutes before slicing and serving.

- **Tips:**
  - For a lighter version, you can substitute half of the eggs with egg whites.
  - Add a sprinkle of red pepper flakes for a bit of heat if desired.

Sweet Quinoa Bowl with Nuts and Sugar-Free Maple Syrup

Preparation Time: 10 minutes, **Cooking Time:** 20 minutes, **Servings:** 4

Ingredients:

- 1 cup quinoa, rinsed
- 2 cups water
- 1/2 tsp cinnamon
- 1/4 cup chopped nuts (almonds, walnuts, or pecans)
- 1/4 cup sugar-free maple syrup (made with xylitol or erythritol)
- Fresh berries for topping (strawberries, blueberries, or raspberries)
- Optional: a sprinkle of chia seeds or flaxseeds for extra fiber

- Nutritional Values:

Nutrient	Per Serving
Calories	240 kcal
Protein	6 g
Carbohydrates	35 g
Fats	8 g
Dietary Fiber	5 g

Procedure:

1. In a medium saucepan, combine rinsed quinoa and water. Bring to a boil, then reduce heat to low, cover, and simmer for 15 minutes or until the water is absorbed.

2. Remove from heat and let it sit covered for 5 minutes. Fluff with a fork and stir in cinnamon.

3. Divide the cooked quinoa into bowls. Top each bowl with chopped nuts and a generous drizzle of sugar-free maple syrup.

4. Add fresh berries and optional chia or flaxseeds on top before serving.

- Tips:
  - To enhance the nutty flavor of the quinoa, toast it in a dry skillet for a few minutes before boiling.
  - This bowl can be served warm or cold, making it versatile for any season.

Nutritious Lunches

Lettuce Wraps with Smoked Turkey, Avocado, and Tahini Sauce

Preparation Time: 15 minutes, **Servings:** 4

Ingredients:

- 8 large lettuce leaves (such as Bibb or Romaine)
- 1 lb smoked turkey breast, thinly sliced
- 1 ripe avocado, sliced
- 1/2 cup shredded carrots
- 1/4 cup red onion, thinly sliced
- **For the tahini sauce:**
  - 1/4 cup tahini
  - 2 tbsp lemon juice
  - 1 clove garlic, minced
  - Salt and pepper to taste
  - Water, as needed to thin the sauce

- **Nutritional Values:**

Nutrient	Per Serving
Calories	250 kcal
Protein	24 g
Carbohydrates	10 g
Fats	14 g
Dietary Fiber	4 g

Procedure:

1. Wash the lettuce leaves gently, pat dry, and set aside.
2. In a small bowl, whisk together the tahini, lemon juice, minced garlic, and season with salt and pepper. Add water a tablespoon at a time until the desired consistency is reached; it should be creamy but pourable.
3. Arrange two lettuce leaves on each plate. Top each leaf with sliced turkey, avocado slices, shredded carrots, and sliced red onion.
4. Drizzle each wrap generously with tahini sauce.

- **Tips:**
  - For added crunch, include sliced cucumbers or chopped nuts in the wraps.
  - These wraps can be prepped ahead of time, but add the tahini sauce just before serving to keep the lettuce crisp.

Reimagined Cobb Salad with Kale, Eggs, and Turkey Bacon

Preparation Time: 20 minutes, **Servings:** 4

Ingredients:

- 4 cups kale, stems removed and leaves chopped
- 4 hard-boiled eggs, peeled and quartered
- 8 slices turkey bacon, cooked and crumbled
- 1 cup cherry tomatoes, halved
- 1 avocado, diced
- 1/2 cup blue cheese, crumbled (optional)
- 1/4 cup red onion, thinly sliced
- **For the dressing:**
  - 1/4 cup olive oil
  - 2 tbsp red wine vinegar
  - 1 tsp Dijon mustard
  - 1 clove garlic, minced
  - Salt and pepper to taste

- Nutritional Values:

Nutrient	Per Serving
Calories	330 kcal
Protein	22 g
Carbohydrates	12 g
Fats	24 g
Dietary Fiber	5 g

Procedure:

1. In a large mixing bowl, add the chopped kale.

2. In a small bowl or jar, combine the olive oil, red wine vinegar, Dijon mustard, minced garlic, salt, and pepper. Whisk or shake until well blended.

3. Pour the dressing over the kale and massage it into the leaves until the kale begins to soften and wilt.

4. Add the quartered eggs, crumbled turkey bacon, halved cherry tomatoes, diced avocado, crumbled blue cheese (if using), and sliced red onion to the kale.

5. Toss gently to combine all ingredients evenly.

6. Serve immediately, ensuring each serving gets an equal share of eggs, bacon, and avocado.

- Tips:
  - For best results, let the dressed kale sit for about 10 minutes before adding the rest of the ingredients; this allows the leaves to become more tender.
  - You can swap turkey bacon for grilled chicken or omit the blue cheese to cater to different dietary preferences.

Tomato and Ginger Soup with Avocado Cream

Preparation Time: 15 minutes, **Cooking Time:** 30 minutes, **Servings:** 4

Ingredients:

- 2 tbsp olive oil
- 1 onion, chopped
- 2 cloves garlic, minced
- 2 tbsp fresh ginger, minced
- 4 cups ripe tomatoes, chopped or 1 (28-ounce) can of whole tomatoes with juice
- 4 cups vegetable broth
- Salt and pepper to taste
- **For the Avocado Cream:**
    - 1 ripe avocado
    - 1/4 cup Greek yogurt
    - Juice of 1 lime
    - Salt to taste

- Nutritional Values:

Nutrient	Per Serving
Calories	200 kcal
Protein	4 g
Carbohydrates	20 g
Fats	12 g
Dietary Fiber	6 g

Procedure:

1. Heat the olive oil in a large pot over medium heat. Add the chopped onion and sauté until translucent, about 5 minutes.
2. Add the minced garlic and ginger, sautéing for another 2 minutes until fragrant.
3. Stir in the chopped tomatoes and cook for a few minutes before pouring in the vegetable broth. Bring the mixture to a boil, then reduce the heat and simmer for 20 minutes.
4. While the soup simmers, prepare the avocado cream by blending the ripe avocado, Greek yogurt, lime juice, and salt until smooth and creamy.
5. After the soup has simmered, use an immersion blender to purée the soup until smooth. Season with salt and pepper.
6. Serve the hot soup with a dollop of avocado cream on top.

- Tips:
    - For a richer flavor, roast the tomatoes in the oven with a drizzle of olive oil before adding them to the soup.
    - The avocado cream can also be used as a spread or dip for other dishes.

Cauliflower 'Rice' Salad with Peas, Carrots, and Almond Sauce

Preparation Time: 20 minutes, **Servings:** 4

Ingredients:

- 1 large head cauliflower, riced
- 1 cup peas, fresh or frozen and thawed
- 1 cup carrots, julienned
- 1/2 cup almonds, slivered
- 2 tbsp olive oil
- For the Almond Sauce:
  - 1/4 cup almond butter
  - 2 tbsp soy sauce (or tamari for gluten-free option)
  - 1 tbsp sesame oil
  - 1 tbsp honey or maple syrup
  - 1 clove garlic, minced
  - 2 tsp ginger, grated
  - Water to thin, as needed

- Nutritional Values:

Nutrient	Per Serving
Calories	280 kcal
Protein	8 g
Carbohydrates	18 g
Fats	20 g
Dietary Fiber	6 g

Procedure:

1. Heat olive oil in a large skillet over medium heat. Add the riced cauliflower and sauté for 5-7 minutes, or until it begins to soften.

2. Add the peas and carrots to the skillet. Continue to cook for another 5 minutes, until all vegetables are tender but still have a bit of crunch.

3. In a small bowl, whisk together almond butter, soy sauce, sesame oil, honey, minced garlic, and grated ginger. Add water a tablespoon at a time until the sauce reaches a pourable consistency.

4. Toss the vegetables in the skillet with the almond sauce until everything is well coated.

5. Garnish with slivered almonds before serving.

- Tips:
  - For a crunchier texture, add the peas and carrots towards the end of the cauliflower cooking time.
  - You can chill the salad for an hour before serving to enhance the flavors.

Lettuce Tacos with Bison Meat and Cilantro Salsa

Preparation Time: 20 minutes, **Cooking Time:** 10 minutes, **Servings:** 4

Ingredients:

- 1 lb ground bison meat
- 8 large lettuce leaves (such as Bibb or Butter lettuce)
- 1 medium onion, diced
- 2 cloves garlic, minced
- 1 tsp ground cumin
- 1 tsp chili powder
- 1/2 tsp salt
- 1/2 tsp black pepper
- **For the Cilantro Salsa:**
    - 1 cup fresh cilantro, chopped
    - 1 tomato, diced
    - 1 jalapeño, seeded and finely chopped
    - Juice of 1 lime
    - Salt to taste

- **Nutritional Values:**

Nutrient	Per Serving
Calories	240 kcal
Protein	21 g
Carbohydrates	6 g
Fats	15 g
Dietary Fiber	2 g

Procedure:

1. In a skillet over medium heat, cook the diced onion and minced garlic until they become translucent, about 3-5 minutes.

2. Add the ground bison meat to the skillet, breaking it up with a spoon. Season with cumin, chili powder, salt, and black pepper. Cook until the meat is browned and fully cooked through, about 5-7 minutes.

3. While the meat cooks, prepare the cilantro salsa by combining the chopped cilantro, diced tomato, finely chopped jalapeño, and lime juice in a bowl. Season with salt and adjust to taste.

4. Assemble the tacos by spooning the cooked bison meat into the lettuce leaves, topped with a generous amount of cilantro salsa.

- **Tips:**
    - For added flavor, you can incorporate a splash of apple cider vinegar or a pinch of smoked paprika into the bison meat as it cooks.
    - If you prefer a milder salsa, substitute the jalapeño with diced green bell pepper.

Cauliflower Rice Bowl with Spicy Shrimp and Lime Sauce

Preparation Time: 15 minutes, **Cooking Time:** 15 minutes, **Servings:** 4

Ingredients:

- 1 large head cauliflower, riced
- 1 lb shrimp, peeled and deveined
- 2 tbsp olive oil
- 1 tsp chili powder
- 1/2 tsp garlic powder
- 1/2 tsp salt
- 1/4 tsp black pepper
- 1 red bell pepper, diced
- 1 cup corn kernels, fresh or frozen
- For the Lime Sauce:
    - 1/4 cup fresh lime juice
    - 2 tbsp honey
    - 1 clove garlic, minced
    - 1 tbsp soy sauce
    - 1 tsp sriracha or another hot sauce (adjust based on heat preference)

- **Nutritional Values:**

Nutrient	Per Serving
Calories	250 kcal
Protein	24 g
Carbohydrates	18 g
Fats	10 g
Dietary Fiber	4 g

Procedure:

1. Heat 1 tablespoon of olive oil in a large skillet over medium heat. Add the riced cauliflower, season with salt and pepper, and sauté for 5-7 minutes until tender. Remove from heat and set aside.

2. In the same skillet, add the remaining tablespoon of olive oil. Toss the shrimp with chili powder, garlic powder, salt, and black pepper, and cook over medium-high heat for 2-3 minutes per side or until pink and cooked through.

3. Add the diced red bell pepper and corn to the skillet with the shrimp during the last 3 minutes of cooking, allowing them to soften slightly.

4. For the lime sauce, whisk together lime juice, honey, minced garlic, soy sauce, and sriracha in a small bowl.

5. To assemble, divide the cauliflower rice among bowls, top with the spicy shrimp, red bell pepper, and corn. Drizzle generously with lime sauce.

- **Tips:**
    - For a complete meal, add some sliced avocado or a handful of fresh cilantro to each bowl before serving. If you prefer a non-spicy version, omit the sriracha and add a pinch of sweet paprika instead.

Kale Salad with Berries, Nuts, and Honey Vinaigrette

Preparation Time: 15 minutes, **Servings:** 4

Ingredients:

- 4 cups kale, stems removed and leaves chopped
- 1 cup mixed berries (blueberries, strawberries, raspberries)
- 1/2 cup nuts (such as almonds or walnuts), toasted
- 1/4 cup feta cheese, crumbled (optional)
- For the Honey Vinaigrette:
    - 1/4 cup olive oil
    - 2 tbsp apple cider vinegar
    - 1 tbsp honey
    - 1 tsp Dijon mustard
    - Salt and pepper to taste

- Nutritional Values:

Nutrient	Per Serving
Calories	280 kcal
Protein	6 g
Carbohydrates	18 g
Fats	21 g
Dietary Fiber	4 g

Procedure:

1. In a large mixing bowl, add the chopped kale. Drizzle a bit of olive oil and a pinch of salt over the kale, then massage the leaves with your hands for about 2 minutes to soften them.

2. Add the mixed berries and toasted nuts to the kale.

3. In a small bowl, whisk together the olive oil, apple cider vinegar, honey, Dijon mustard, salt, and pepper to make the vinaigrette.

4. Pour the vinaigrette over the salad and toss well to coat all the ingredients evenly.

5. If using, sprinkle the crumbled feta cheese over the salad just before serving.

- Tips:
    - Massaging the kale helps to break down its fibers and soften the leaves, making them easier to eat and digest.
    - For a protein boost, consider adding grilled chicken or salmon to the salad

Turkey Chili with Black Beans and Avocado

Preparation Time: 20 minutes, **Cooking Time:** 1 hour, **Servings:** 6

Ingredients:

- 1 tbsp olive oil
- 1 lb ground turkey
- 1 large onion, diced
- 2 cloves garlic, minced
- 1 red bell pepper, diced
- 1 can (15 oz) black beans, drained and rinsed
- 1 can (28 oz) diced tomatoes
- 2 cups chicken broth
- 2 tbsp chili powder
- 1 tbsp ground cumin
- 1 tsp smoked paprika
- Salt and black pepper to taste
- 1 ripe avocado, diced
- Fresh cilantro, chopped, for garnish

- **Nutritional Values:**

Nutrient	Per Serving
Calories	300 kcal
Protein	23 g
Carbohydrates	25 g
Fats	12 g
Dietary Fiber	7 g

Procedure:

1. Heat the olive oil in a large pot over medium heat. Add the ground turkey and cook until browned, breaking it up with a spoon as it cooks.

2. Add the diced onion, garlic, and red bell pepper to the pot. Sauté until the vegetables are tender, about 5 minutes.

3. Stir in the black beans, diced tomatoes, chicken broth, chili powder, ground cumin, and smoked paprika. Season with salt and black pepper.

4. Bring the mixture to a boil, then reduce the heat to low and simmer, uncovered, for about 45 minutes, stirring occasionally.

5. Once the chili has thickened and the flavors have melded together, remove from heat.

6. Serve the chili in bowls, topped with diced avocado and chopped cilantro.

- **Tips:**
  - For a spicier chili, add a diced jalapeño or a teaspoon of cayenne pepper during the cooking process.
  - This chili can be stored in the refrigerator for up to 3 days or frozen for longer storage. The flavors often improve the next day.

Vegetable Skewers with Tahini and Lemon Sauce

Preparation Time: 15 minutes, **Cooking Time:** 10 minutes, **Servings:** 4

Ingredients:

- 2 zucchinis, sliced into rounds
- 2 red bell peppers, cut into chunks
- 1 large red onion, cut into wedges
- 1 pint cherry tomatoes
- 2 tbsp olive oil
- Salt and black pepper to taste
- **For the Tahini and Lemon Sauce:**
    - 1/4 cup tahini
    - 1/4 cup water
    - Juice of 1 lemon
    - 1 clove garlic, minced
    - Salt to taste

- Nutritional Values:

Nutrient	Per Serving
Calories	180 kcal
Protein	4 g
Carbohydrates	18 g
Fats	12 g
Dietary Fiber	4 g

Procedure:

1. Preheat your grill to medium-high heat.
2. Thread the sliced zucchinis, red bell peppers, red onions, and cherry tomatoes onto skewers. Brush them with olive oil and season with salt and black pepper.
3. Grill the skewers, turning occasionally, until the vegetables are tender and charred in spots, about 8-10 minutes.
4. While the skewers are grilling, prepare the tahini and lemon sauce by whisking together tahini, water, lemon juice, minced garlic, and salt in a bowl until smooth and creamy.
5. Serve the grilled vegetable skewers drizzled with the tahini and lemon sauce.

- Tips:
    - If using wooden skewers, soak them in water for at least 30 minutes prior to grilling to prevent burning.
    - This dish can be served as a side or paired with a protein like grilled chicken or fish for a more substantial meal.

Tandoori Chicken with Cucumber Salad and Greek Yogurt

Preparation Time: 20 minutes (plus marinating time), **Cooking Time:** 30 minutes, **Servings:** 4

Ingredients:

- 4 boneless, skinless chicken breasts
- 1 cup Greek yogurt (for marinade)
- 2 tbsp tandoori masala spice blend
- 1 lemon, juiced
- 2 cloves garlic, minced
- 1 tbsp grated ginger
- Salt to taste
- **For the Cucumber Salad:**
  - 2 large cucumbers, thinly sliced
  - 1/4 cup red onion, thinly sliced
  - 1/4 cup Greek yogurt
  - 1 tbsp lemon juice
  - 1 tbsp fresh dill, chopped
  - Salt and pepper to taste
- Additional Greek yogurt for serving

- Nutritional Values:

Nutrient	Per Serving
Calories	310 kcal
Protein	36 g
Carbohydrates	10 g
Fats	14 g
Dietary Fiber	1 g

Procedure:

1. In a bowl, combine the Greek yogurt, tandoori masala, lemon juice, minced garlic, grated ginger, and salt. Add the chicken breasts and coat them thoroughly with the marinade. Cover and refrigerate for at least 2 hours, or overnight for best flavor.

2. Preheat your grill or oven to 400°F (200°C). If grilling, place the chicken on the grill and cook for about 5-7 minutes on each side, or until fully cooked. If baking, place the chicken in a baking dish and bake for about 20-25 minutes, or until the chicken is cooked through and the juices run clear.

3. While the chicken cooks, prepare the cucumber salad by combining the sliced cucumbers, red onion, Greek yogurt, lemon juice, fresh dill, salt, and pepper in a bowl. Mix well and refrigerate until ready to serve.

4. Serve the cooked chicken with a side of cucumber salad and a dollop of Greek yogurt.

- Tips:
  - Ensure the chicken is marinated long enough to absorb the flavors fully, ideally overnight.
  - For an authentic charred tandoori look, you can briefly broil the chicken after baking.

Lettuce Wraps with Lamb Meatballs and Tzatziki Sauce

Preparation Time: 30 minutes, **Cooking Time:** 20 minutes, **Servings:** 4

Ingredients:

- For the Lamb Meatballs:
    - 1 lb ground lamb
    - 1 small onion, finely grated
    - 2 cloves garlic, minced
    - 1/4 cup fresh parsley, finely chopped
    - 1 tsp ground cumin
    - 1 tsp paprika
    - 1/2 tsp salt
    - 1/4 tsp black pepper
- For the Tzatziki Sauce:
    - 1 cup Greek yogurt
    - 1/2 cucumber, seeded and finely grated
    - 2 tbsp lemon juice
    - 1 tbsp olive oil
    - 1 clove garlic, minced
    - 1 tbsp fresh dill, chopped
    - Salt and pepper to taste
- Large lettuce leaves (such as Bibb or Romaine), for serving
- Optional garnishes: diced tomatoes, sliced cucumbers, red onion slices

- Nutritional Values:

Nutrient	Per Serving
Calories	320 kcal
Protein	23 g
Carbohydrates	8 g
Fats	22 g
Dietary Fiber	1 g

Procedure:

1. Preheat the oven to 375°F (190°C).

2. In a bowl, combine the ground lamb, grated onion, minced garlic, chopped parsley, cumin, paprika, salt, and pepper. Mix until well combined.

3. Form the mixture into small, bite-sized meatballs and place them on a baking sheet lined with parchment paper.

4. Bake the meatballs for about 15-20 minutes, or until they are cooked through and slightly browned on the outside.

5. While the meatballs bake, prepare the tzatziki sauce by combining the Greek yogurt, grated cucumber, lemon juice, olive oil, minced garlic, chopped dill, salt, and pepper in a bowl. Stir until well mixed and refrigerate until ready to use. To serve, place a few meatballs in each lettuce leaf, top with tzatziki sauce, and add optional garnishes like diced tomatoes, sliced cucumbers, or red onion slices.

Chickpea and Avocado Salad with Lime and Cilantro

Preparation Time: 15 minutes, **Servings:** 4

Ingredients:

- 1 can (15 oz) chickpeas, rinsed and drained
- 2 ripe avocados, diced
- 1 red onion, finely chopped
- 1 cup cherry tomatoes, halved
- 1/4 cup fresh cilantro, chopped
- Juice of 2 limes
- 2 tbsp olive oil
- Salt and pepper to taste
- Optional: 1 jalapeño, seeded and finely chopped

- **Nutritional Values:**

Nutrient	Per Serving
Calories	300 kcal
Protein	8 g
Carbohydrates	32 g
Fats	18 g
Dietary Fiber	10 g

Procedure:

1. In a large bowl, combine the chickpeas, diced avocados, chopped red onion, halved cherry tomatoes, and chopped cilantro.

2. In a small bowl, whisk together the lime juice, olive oil, salt, and pepper. If using, add the chopped jalapeño to the dressing for a spicy kick.

3. Pour the dressing over the salad ingredients and gently toss to coat everything evenly.

4. Adjust seasoning with additional salt and pepper if needed.

- **Tips:**
    - For the best flavor, let the salad sit for about 10 minutes before serving to allow the flavors to meld.
    - This salad is very versatile; add cooked quinoa or feta cheese for extra protein and texture.

Zoodles (Zucchini Noodles) with Cashew Alfredo Sauce

Preparation Time: 15 minutes, **Cooking Time:** 10 minutes, **Servings:** 4

Ingredients:

- 4 medium zucchini, spiralized or cut into noodles
- 1 cup raw cashews, soaked in water for 4 hours or overnight, then drained
- 1 cup unsweetened almond milk
- 2 cloves garlic, minced
- 2 tbsp nutritional yeast
- 1 tbsp lemon juice
- 1/2 tsp salt
- 1/4 tsp black pepper
- Optional: pinch of nutmeg
- Fresh parsley, chopped, for garnish

- **Nutritional Values:**

Nutrient	Per Serving
Calories	220 kcal
Protein	8 g
Carbohydrates	18 g
Fats	14 g
Dietary Fiber	4 g

Procedure:

1. Prepare the zucchini noodles using a spiralizer or a vegetable peeler and set them aside.

2. In a blender, combine the soaked and drained cashews, almond milk, minced garlic, nutritional yeast, lemon juice, salt, and black pepper. Blend until smooth and creamy. Adjust the consistency by adding a little more almond milk if necessary.

3. Heat a large skillet over medium heat. Add the cashew Alfredo sauce and warm it gently, stirring frequently to prevent sticking. If desired, add a pinch of nutmeg.

4. Add the zucchini noodles to the skillet and toss with the sauce for about 2-3 minutes, just until the noodles are heated through but still firm.

5. Serve the zoodles garnished with chopped fresh parsley.

- **Tips:**
  - Avoid overcooking the zucchini noodles to prevent them from becoming too soft or watery.
  - For added protein, top the zoodles with grilled chicken or sautéed shrimp.

Tuna Salad with Celery, Red Onions, and Greek Yogurt

Preparation Time: 10 minutes, **Servings:** 4

Ingredients:

- 2 cans (each 5 oz) tuna in water, drained
- 1/2 cup Greek yogurt
- 1/4 cup celery, finely chopped
- 1/4 cup red onion, finely chopped
- 1 tbsp lemon juice
- 1 tbsp fresh parsley, chopped
- Salt and pepper to taste
- Optional: 1 tsp Dijon mustard for extra flavor

- **Nutritional Values:**

Nutrient	Per Serving
Calories	120 kcal
Protein	20 g
Carbohydrates	3 g
Fats	2 g
Dietary Fiber	1 g

Procedure:

1. In a medium bowl, mix together the drained tuna, Greek yogurt, finely chopped celery, finely chopped red onion, lemon juice, and chopped parsley. If using, add the Dijon mustard.

2. Season the salad with salt and pepper to taste. Stir well until all ingredients are evenly combined.

3. Refrigerate the salad for at least 30 minutes before serving to allow the flavors to meld together.

- **Tips:**
    - Serve this tuna salad on whole-grain bread for a healthy sandwich or over a bed of lettuce for a low-carb option.
    - You can add chopped hard-boiled eggs or capers for additional texture and flavor.

Lettuce Wraps with Hummus, Cucumbers and Kalamata Olives

Preparation Time: 10 minutes, **Servings:** 4

Ingredients:

- 8 large lettuce leaves (such as Bibb or Romaine)
- 1 cup hummus
- 1 cucumber, thinly sliced
- 1/2 cup Kalamata olives, pitted and sliced
- Optional garnishes: diced tomatoes, red onion slices, feta cheese, fresh parsley

- Nutritional Values:

Nutrient	Per Serving
Calories	150 kcal
Protein	5 g
Carbohydrates	13 g
Fats	9 g
Dietary Fiber	3 g

Procedure:

1. Carefully rinse and dry the lettuce leaves, then lay them out on a clean surface.
2. Spread about 2 tablespoons of hummus on each lettuce leaf.
3. Top the hummus with several slices of cucumber and a sprinkling of sliced Kalamata olives.
4. If desired, add additional garnishes like diced tomatoes, red onion slices, crumbled feta cheese, or a sprinkle of fresh parsley.
5. Carefully fold or roll the lettuce leaves to enclose the fillings, creating wraps.

- Tips:
    - For a protein boost, consider adding grilled chicken strips or chickpeas to the wraps.
    - These wraps are best enjoyed fresh but can be prepped a few hours ahead if kept in the fridge.

Healthy and Tasty Dinners

Roast Chicken with Avocado Chimichurri Sauce

Preparation Time: 20 minutes, **Cooking Time:** 1 hour, **Servings:** 4

Ingredients:

- **For the Roast Chicken:**
  - 1 whole chicken (about 4-5 lbs)
  - 2 tbsp olive oil
  - 1 tsp salt
  - 1/2 tsp black pepper
  - 1/2 tsp paprika
  - 1/2 tsp garlic powder
  - Fresh herbs (like rosemary or thyme), optional

- **For the Avocado Chimichurri Sauce:**
  - 1 ripe avocado, pitted and peeled
  - 1/2 cup fresh parsley, chopped
  - 1/4 cup fresh cilantro, chopped
  - 3 cloves garlic, minced
  - 2 tbsp red wine vinegar
  - 1/2 cup olive oil
  - 1 tbsp lime juice
  - Salt and pepper to taste
  - Red pepper flakes, optional

- Nutritional Values:

Nutrient	Per Serving
Calories	450 kcal
Protein	35 g
Carbohydrates	6 g
Fats	34 g
Dietary Fiber	3 g

Procedure:

1. Preheat your oven to 400°F (200°C). Pat the chicken dry with paper towels. Rub the chicken all over with olive oil and season generously with salt, pepper, paprika, and garlic powder. If using, stuff the cavity with fresh herbs.

2. Place the chicken in a roasting pan and roast for about 1 hour or until the internal temperature reaches 165°F (74°C) and the skin is golden and crisp.

3. While the chicken roasts, make the chimichurri sauce. In a food processor, combine the avocado, parsley, cilantro, garlic, red wine vinegar, olive oil, and lime juice. Pulse until smooth. Season with salt, pepper, and red pepper flakes if desired. Let the chicken rest for 10 minutes after roasting. Serve it sliced with a generous drizzle of the avocado chimichurri sauce.

Sesame-Crusted Salmon Bowl with Kale and Tamari Soy Sauce

Preparation Time: 15 minutes, **Cooking Time:** 20 minutes, **Servings:** 4

Ingredients:

- For the Sesame-Crusted Salmon:
  - 4 salmon fillets (about 6 oz each)
  - 2 tbsp sesame oil
  - 1/4 cup white sesame seeds
  - 1/4 cup black sesame seeds
  - Salt and black pepper to taste
- For the Kale and Tamari Soy Sauce:
  - 2 tbsp olive oil
  - 4 cups chopped kale
  - 2 tbsp tamari soy sauce
  - 2 cloves garlic, minced
  - 1 tbsp ginger, grated
  - Optional: red pepper flakes
- For Garnish:
  - Sliced green onions
  - Sliced avocado

- **Nutritional Values:**

Nutrient	Per Serving
Calories	390 kcal
Protein	34 g
Carbohydrates	10 g
Fats	25 g
Dietary Fiber	4 g

Procedure:

1. Preheat your oven to 400°F (200°C).

2. Mix white and black sesame seeds on a plate, seasoning with a little salt and pepper. Press each salmon fillet into the sesame seed mixture, coating both sides.

3. Heat sesame oil in a skillet over medium-high heat. Add the salmon fillets and sear each side for about 2 minutes until golden. Transfer the skillet to the oven and bake the salmon for an additional 10 minutes, or until cooked through and flaky.

4. While the salmon is cooking, heat olive oil in another skillet over medium heat. Add garlic and ginger, sautéing for about 1 minute until fragrant. Add the kale and tamari soy sauce, cooking until the kale is wilted and tender. Sprinkle with red pepper flakes if using.

5. To assemble the bowls, divide the sautéed kale among four bowls. Place a salmon fillet in each bowl. Garnish with sliced green onions and avocado.

Tips: Ensure the sesame seeds adhere well to the salmon by pressing them gently with your hands. The kale can be replaced with other hearty greens like Swiss chard or spinach if desired.

Oven-Baked Pork Ribs with Coconut Pineapple BBQ Sauce

Preparation Time: 20 minutes (plus marinating time), **Cooking Time:** 2 hours, **Servings:** 4

Ingredients:

- For the Pork Ribs:
    - 2 racks of pork ribs (about 3 lbs each)
    - 2 tbsp paprika
    - 1 tbsp garlic powder
    - 1 tbsp onion powder
    - 1 tbsp ground cumin
    - 1 tbsp salt
    - 1 tbsp black pepper
- For the Coconut Pineapple BBQ Sauce:
    - 1 cup pineapple juice
    - 1/2 cup coconut milk
    - 1/4 cup apple cider vinegar
    - 1/4 cup brown sugar
    - 2 tbsp soy sauce
    - 1 tbsp fresh ginger, grated
    - 2 cloves garlic, minced
    - 1 tsp chili flakes (optional)

- Nutritional Values:

Nutrient	Per Serving
Calories	780 kcal
Protein	64 g
Carbohydrates	20 g
Fats	50 g
Dietary Fiber	1 g

Procedure:

1. Preheat your oven to 300°F (150°C).

2. In a small bowl, combine paprika, garlic powder, onion powder, ground cumin, salt, and black pepper. Rub this mixture all over the ribs, covering all sides. Place the ribs on a baking sheet lined with aluminum foil, and cover with another piece of foil. Bake for about 1.5 to 2 hours, or until the meat is tender and falls off the bone.

3. While the ribs are baking, make the BBQ sauce. Combine pineapple juice, coconut milk, apple cider vinegar, brown sugar, soy sauce, grated ginger, minced garlic, and chili flakes in a saucepan over medium heat. Bring to a simmer and cook until the sauce thickens, about 20 minutes.

4. Remove the ribs from the oven and discard the top piece of foil. Brush the ribs generously with the coconut pineapple BBQ sauce and return to the oven, uncovered, for an additional 20-30 minutes to caramelize the sauce.

5. Serve the ribs with extra BBQ sauce on the side.

Tips: For deeper flavor, you can marinate the ribs with the dry rub overnight in the refrigerator before baking.

Nut-Crusted Cod Fillet with Roasted Asparagus

Preparation Time: 15 minutes, **Cooking Time:** 20 minutes, **Servings:** 4

Ingredients:

- **For the Nut-Crusted Cod:**
    - 4 cod fillets (about 6 oz each)
    - 1/2 cup mixed nuts (almonds, pecans, walnuts), finely chopped
    - 2 tbsp olive oil
    - 1 tbsp lemon zest
    - Salt and pepper to taste
- **For the Roasted Asparagus:**
    - 1 lb asparagus, trimmed
    - 2 tbsp olive oil
    - Salt and pepper to taste
    - Lemon wedges, for serving

- **Nutritional Values:**

Nutrient	Per Serving
Calories	360 kcal
Protein	28 g
Carbohydrates	8 g
Fats	24 g
Dietary Fiber	3 g

Procedure:

1. Preheat your oven to 400°F (200°C).
2. Place the finely chopped nuts in a shallow dish, mix in the lemon zest, and season with salt and pepper.
3. Brush each cod fillet lightly with olive oil, then press into the nut mixture to coat the top side of each fillet.
4. Arrange the nut-crusted cod fillets on a lined baking tray.
5. Toss the asparagus with olive oil, salt, and pepper, and spread them around the cod on the baking tray.
6. Bake in the preheated oven for about 15-20 minutes, or until the cod is cooked through and the nuts are golden brown.
7. Serve the nut-crusted cod and roasted asparagus with lemon wedges on the side.

Tips: Make sure the nuts are finely chopped to create a uniform crust that adheres well to the cod. For extra flavor, sprinkle garlic powder or Parmesan cheese over the asparagus before roasting.

Beef and Cauliflower 'Barley' Soup with Roasted Vegetables

Preparation Time: 20 minutes, **Cooking Time:** 1 hour, **Servings:** 6

Ingredients:

- For the Roasted Vegetables:
  - 1 cup cauliflower florets
  - 1 cup carrots, diced
  - 1 cup parsnips, diced
  - 2 tbsp olive oil
  - Salt and pepper to taste
- For the Soup:
  - 1 lb beef stew meat, cut into cubes
  - 2 tbsp olive oil
  - 1 onion, chopped
  - 2 cloves garlic, minced
  - 6 cups beef broth
  - 1/2 cup chopped celery
  - 1 tsp dried thyme
  - 1 bay leaf
  - Salt and pepper to taste

- Nutritional Values:

Nutrient	Per Serving
Calories	300 kcal
Protein	24 g
Carbohydrates	15 g
Fats	16 g
Dietary Fiber	4 g

Procedure:

1. Preheat the oven to 400°F (200°C). Toss the cauliflower, carrots, and parsnips with olive oil, salt, and pepper. Spread on a baking sheet and roast for 30 minutes, or until vegetables are golden and tender.

2. While the vegetables are roasting, heat olive oil in a large pot over medium-high heat. Add the beef cubes and brown on all sides. Remove the beef and set aside.

3. In the same pot, add the chopped onion and garlic, sautéing until the onion becomes translucent.

4. Return the beef to the pot, add beef broth, celery, thyme, and bay leaf. Bring to a boil, then reduce heat to a simmer. Cover and cook for about 30 minutes.

5. Add the roasted vegetables to the pot and continue to simmer for an additional 10 minutes. Adjust seasoning with salt and pepper.

6. Remove the bay leaf before serving.

Tips: Roasting the vegetables before adding them to the soup enhances their flavor and adds a rich depth to the dish. For a thicker soup, you can puree a portion of the cooked vegetables and stir them back into the pot.

Turkey Burgers with Guacamole and Baked Sweet Potato Fries

Preparation Time: 20 minutes, **Cooking Time:** 30 minutes, **Servings:** 4

Ingredients:

- For the Turkey Burgers:
    - 1 lb ground turkey
    - 1/4 cup breadcrumbs
    - 1 egg
    - 2 cloves garlic, minced
    - 1 tsp smoked paprika
    - 1 tsp salt
    - 1/2 tsp black pepper
- For the Guacamole:
    - 2 ripe avocados
    - 1 small onion, finely chopped
    - 1 tomato, diced
    - Juice of 1 lime
    - Salt and pepper to taste
- For the Sweet Potato Fries:
    - 2 large sweet potatoes, peeled and cut into fries
    - 2 tbsp olive oil
    - 1 tsp paprika
    - Salt to taste

- **Nutritional Values:**

Nutrient	Per Serving
Calories	470 kcal
Protein	28 g
Carbohydrates	45 g
Fats	22 g
Dietary Fiber	8 g

Procedure:

1. **For the Sweet Potato Fries:** Preheat the oven to 400°F (200°C). Toss the sweet potato fries with olive oil, paprika, and salt. Spread on a baking sheet in a single layer. Bake for 25-30 minutes, turning halfway through, until crispy and golden.

2. **For the Turkey Burgers:** In a bowl, mix together the ground turkey, breadcrumbs, egg, minced garlic, smoked paprika, salt, and pepper. Form into 4 patties. Heat a grill pan or skillet over medium heat and cook the patties for about 5-6 minutes per side, or until fully cooked.

3. **For the Guacamole:** In a bowl, mash the avocados. Mix in the chopped onion, diced tomato, lime juice, salt, and pepper.

4. **To Serve:** Serve each turkey burger with a generous scoop of guacamole and a side of baked sweet potato fries.

Tips: Make sure not to overcrowd the pan when cooking the burgers to ensure they get a nice sear.

Baked Eggplant and Tomato Casserole with Almond Mozzarella

Preparation Time: 20 minutes, **Cooking Time:** 40 minutes, **Servings:** 4

Ingredients:

- For the Casserole:
    - 2 large eggplants, sliced into 1/2-inch thick rounds
    - 3 large tomatoes, sliced
    - 1/2 cup almond mozzarella, grated
    - 1/4 cup fresh basil leaves, chopped
    - 2 cloves garlic, minced
    - 2 tbsp olive oil
    - Salt and pepper to taste
- For the Almond Mozzarella:
    - 1 cup blanched almonds, soaked overnight
    - 1/4 cup water
    - 2 tbsp nutritional yeast
    - 1 tbsp lemon juice
    - 1/2 tsp salt

- Nutritional Values:

Nutrient	Per Serving
Calories	300 kcal
Protein	10 g
Carbohydrates	23 g
Fats	20 g
Dietary Fiber	11 g

Procedure:

1. **For the Almond Mozzarella:**
   - Drain and rinse the soaked almonds. Blend almonds with water, nutritional yeast, lemon juice, and salt in a high-speed blender until smooth and creamy. Adjust consistency by adding more water if needed.

2. Preheat the oven to 375°F (190°C).

3. Brush each eggplant slice with olive oil and season with salt and pepper. Arrange a layer of eggplant slices at the bottom of a baking dish.

4. Layer tomato slices over the eggplant, sprinkle with minced garlic, and some of the basil. Repeat the layering until all ingredients are used up.

5. Top the final layer with almond mozzarella. Cover with foil and bake for 30 minutes. Remove the foil and bake for another 10 minutes, or until the cheese is golden and bubbly.

6. Garnish with the remaining basil before serving.

Grilled Fish Tacos with Mango Salsa and Cilantro

Preparation Time: 20 minutes, **Cooking Time:** 10 minutes, **Servings:** 4

Ingredients:

- For the Grilled Fish:
    - 4 tilapia fillets (or any firm white fish)
    - 2 tbsp olive oil
    - 1 tsp chili powder
    - 1 tsp cumin
    - Salt and pepper to taste
- For the Mango Salsa:
    - 1 ripe mango, peeled and diced
    - 1/4 cup red onion, finely chopped
    - 1 jalapeño, seeded and finely chopped
    - 1/4 cup fresh cilantro, chopped
    - Juice of 1 lime
    - Salt to taste
- Additional Ingredients:
    - 8 small corn tortillas
    - Lime wedges for serving

- Nutritional Values:

Nutrient	Per Serving
Calories	350 kcal
Protein	23 g
Carbohydrates	35 g
Fats	12 g
Dietary Fiber	5 g

Procedure:

1. **For the Grilled Fish:**
   - Preheat grill to medium-high heat.
   - Brush the fish fillets with olive oil and season with chili powder, cumin, salt, and pepper.
   - Grill the fish for about 3-4 minutes on each side or until the fish flakes easily with a fork.

2. **For the Mango Salsa:** In a bowl, combine the diced mango, chopped red onion, chopped jalapeño, chopped cilantro, and lime juice. Season with salt and mix well.

3. **To Serve:**
   - Warm the corn tortillas on the grill or in a skillet.
   - Break the grilled fish into pieces and divide among the tortillas.
   - Top each taco with a generous amount of mango salsa.
   - Serve with lime wedges on the side.

Lamb Stew with Root Vegetables and Rosemary

Preparation Time: 20 minutes, **Cooking Time:** 2 hours, **Servings:** 6

Ingredients:

- For the Lamb Stew:
    - 2 lbs lamb shoulder, cut into cubes
    - 2 tbsp olive oil
    - 1 large onion, chopped
    - 3 cloves garlic, minced
    - 3 carrots, peeled and diced
    - 3 parsnips, peeled and diced
    - 2 turnips, peeled and diced
    - 4 cups beef or lamb broth
    - 1 cup red wine
    - 2 tbsp tomato paste
    - 2 sprigs fresh rosemary
    - 2 bay leaves
    - Salt and pepper to taste

- Nutritional Values:

Nutrient	Per Serving
Calories	450 kcal
Protein	35 g
Carbohydrates	20 g
Fats	25 g
Dietary Fiber	5 g

Procedure:

1. Heat olive oil in a large pot or Dutch oven over medium-high heat. Add the lamb cubes and brown on all sides, about 5-7 minutes. Remove the lamb and set aside.

2. In the same pot, add the chopped onion and minced garlic. Cook until the onion is translucent, about 5 minutes.

3. Return the lamb to the pot along with carrots, parsnips, and turnips. Stir to combine.

4. Add the beef or lamb broth, red wine, tomato paste, rosemary sprigs, and bay leaves. Bring to a boil, then reduce the heat to low and simmer covered for about 1.5 to 2 hours, or until the lamb is tender and the vegetables are cooked.

5. Season with salt and pepper to taste. Remove the bay leaves and rosemary sprigs before serving.

Tips:

- For a thicker stew, you can remove a cup of the stew, blend it until smooth, and then stir it back into the pot.
- This stew tastes even better the next day as the flavors have more time to meld together.

Carrot and Curry Soup with Coconut Milk

Preparation Time: 15 minutes, **Cooking Time:** 30 minutes, **Servings:** 4

Ingredients:

- 1 tbsp olive oil
- 1 onion, chopped
- 2 cloves garlic, minced
- 1 tbsp curry powder
- 1 tsp ground ginger
- 1/2 tsp salt
- 1/4 tsp black pepper
- 1 lb carrots, peeled and chopped
- 4 cups vegetable broth
- 1 can (14 oz) coconut milk
- Optional garnishes: chopped cilantro, toasted coconut flakes, a squeeze of lime

- **Nutritional Values:**

Nutrient	Per Serving
Calories	250 kcal
Protein	3 g
Carbohydrates	25 g
Fats	15 g
Dietary Fiber	5 g

Procedure:

1. Heat the olive oil in a large pot over medium heat. Add the chopped onion and sauté until translucent, about 5 minutes.

2. Add the minced garlic, curry powder, and ground ginger, stirring until fragrant, about 1 minute.

3. Add the chopped carrots to the pot and season with salt and pepper. Stir to coat the carrots with the spices.

4. Pour in the vegetable broth and bring the mixture to a boil. Reduce the heat and simmer for about 20 minutes, or until the carrots are very tender.

5. Remove the soup from heat and use an immersion blender to puree the soup until smooth.

6. Stir in the coconut milk and heat through. Adjust seasoning if needed.

7. Serve the soup hot, garnished with chopped cilantro, toasted coconut flakes, and a squeeze of lime if desired.

- Tips:
  - If you don't have an immersion blender, you can carefully transfer the soup in batches to a blender to puree.
  - For an extra layer of flavor, roast the carrots in the oven with a bit of curry powder before adding them to the soup.

Salmon Burgers with Dill and Lemon Sauce

Preparation Time: 15 minutes, **Cooking Time:** 10 minutes, **Servings:** 4

Ingredients:

- For the Salmon Burgers:
  - 1 lb fresh salmon fillet, finely chopped or ground
  - 1/4 cup breadcrumbs
  - 1 egg, beaten
  - 2 tbsp fresh dill, chopped
  - 1 tbsp Dijon mustard
  - 1 tsp lemon zest
  - Salt and pepper to taste
- For the Dill and Lemon Sauce:
  - 1/2 cup Greek yogurt
  - 2 tbsp fresh dill, chopped
  - 1 tbsp lemon juice
  - 1 tsp lemon zest
  - Salt and pepper to taste
- Additional:
  - 4 whole-grain burger buns
  - Lettuce, tomato slices, and onion slices for serving

- **Nutritional Values:**

Nutrient	Per Serving
Calories	380 kcal
Protein	28 g
Carbohydrates	28 g
Fats	18 g
Dietary Fiber	3 g

Procedure:

1. In a bowl, mix together the chopped salmon, breadcrumbs, egg, chopped dill, Dijon mustard, lemon zest, salt, and pepper. Form the mixture into 4 burger patties.

2. Heat a grill pan or skillet over medium heat and lightly oil it. Grill the salmon patties for about 4-5 minutes on each side, or until fully cooked and golden.

3. While the burgers are cooking, prepare the dill and lemon sauce by mixing together the Greek yogurt, chopped dill, lemon juice, lemon zest, salt, and pepper in a small bowl.

4. Toast the burger buns, if desired. Assemble the burgers by placing a salmon patty on each bun, topped with lettuce, tomato slices, onion slices, and a generous dollop of dill and lemon sauce.

- **Tips:**
  - Make sure to chop the salmon finely to help the patties hold together better during cooking.
  - For an extra kick, add a minced clove of garlic to the burger mix or the sauce

Roasted Cauliflower with Tahini and Pomegranate

Preparation Time: 10 minutes, **Cooking Time:** 25 minutes, **Servings:** 4

Ingredients:

- 1 large head of cauliflower, cut into florets
- 2 tbsp olive oil
- Salt and pepper to taste
- **For the Tahini Sauce:**
    - 1/4 cup tahini
    - 2 tbsp lemon juice
    - 1 clove garlic, minced
    - 2-4 tbsp water, as needed for consistency
    - Salt to taste
- **To Garnish:**
    - 1/2 cup pomegranate seeds
    - 2 tbsp chopped fresh parsley

- Nutritional Values:

Nutrient	Per Serving
Calories	210 kcal
Protein	5 g
Carbohydrates	18 g
Fats	14 g
Dietary Fiber	5 g

Procedure:

1. Preheat your oven to 425°F (220°C).
2. Toss the cauliflower florets with olive oil, salt, and pepper. Spread them on a baking sheet in a single layer.
3. Roast in the preheated oven for about 20-25 minutes, or until golden and tender, stirring halfway through cooking.
4. While the cauliflower is roasting, prepare the tahini sauce. In a small bowl, whisk together the tahini, lemon juice, minced garlic, and water until smooth. Season with salt to taste.
5. Once the cauliflower is roasted, transfer it to a serving dish. Drizzle with the tahini sauce, then sprinkle with pomegranate seeds and chopped parsley.

- Tips:
    - Roasting the cauliflower until it is nicely caramelized brings out its natural sweetness and enhances the flavors.
    - The tahini sauce can be prepared in advance and stored in the refrigerator. Give it a quick stir before serving, as it may thicken upon standing.

Almond Flour Pizza with Prosciutto and Arugula

Preparation Time: 15 minutes, **Cooking Time:** 20 minutes, **Servings:** 4

Ingredients:

- For the Pizza Crust:
    - 2 cups almond flour
    - 1 egg
    - 1 tbsp olive oil
    - 1 tsp baking powder
    - 1/2 tsp salt
- Toppings:
    - 1/2 cup tomato sauce
    - 1 cup mozzarella cheese, shredded
    - 4 slices prosciutto, torn into pieces
    - 1 cup arugula
    - 1/2 cup shaved Parmesan cheese
    - Extra virgin olive oil, for drizzling
    - Red pepper flakes (optional)

- Nutritional Values:

Nutrient	Per Serving
Calories	560 kcal
Protein	25 g
Carbohydrates	20 g
Fats	44 g
Dietary Fiber	6 g

Procedure:

1. Preheat your oven to 350°F (175°C).
2. In a bowl, combine almond flour, egg, olive oil, baking powder, and salt. Mix until a dough forms.
3. Place the dough between two pieces of parchment paper and roll out to your desired thickness for a pizza crust.
4. Remove the top parchment paper and transfer the bottom sheet with the dough onto a baking tray.
5. Pre-bake the crust for about 10 minutes, or until it starts to turn golden.
6. Remove from the oven and spread tomato sauce over the crust. Sprinkle with mozzarella cheese and add prosciutto pieces.
7. Return to the oven and bake for another 10 minutes, or until the cheese is melted and bubbly.
8. Top the hot pizza with arugula and shaved Parmesan. Drizzle with extra virgin olive oil and sprinkle red pepper flakes if using.
9. Slice and serve immediately.

Cauliflower Soup with Ginger and Turmeric

Preparation Time: 15 minutes, **Cooking Time:** 30 minutes, **Servings:** 4

Ingredients:

- 1 tbsp olive oil
- 1 onion, chopped
- 2 cloves garlic, minced
- 1 tbsp fresh ginger, grated
- 1 tsp turmeric powder
- 1 head of cauliflower, cut into florets
- 4 cups vegetable broth
- Salt and pepper to taste
- 1 can (14 oz) coconut milk
- Optional garnishes: chopped cilantro, a swirl of coconut cream, toasted almond slices

- **Nutritional Values:**

Nutrient	Per Serving
Calories	220 kcal
Protein	5 g
Carbohydrates	15 g
Fats	16 g
Dietary Fiber	4 g

Procedure:

1. Heat the olive oil in a large pot over medium heat. Add the chopped onion and sauté until translucent, about 5 minutes.

2. Add the minced garlic, grated ginger, and turmeric powder, cooking for another minute until fragrant.

3. Add the cauliflower florets and stir well to coat with the spices.

4. Pour in the vegetable broth, bring to a boil, then reduce to a simmer. Cover and let cook for about 20 minutes or until the cauliflower is tender.

5. Use an immersion blender to puree the soup directly in the pot until smooth. Alternatively, carefully transfer to a blender in batches.

6. Stir in the coconut milk and heat through. Season with salt and pepper to taste.

7. Serve hot, garnished with chopped cilantro, a swirl of coconut cream, and toasted almond slices if desired.

- **Tips:**
    - Adjust the consistency of the soup by adding more vegetable broth if it's too thick or letting it simmer longer if too thin.
    - The addition of turmeric not only gives this soup a beautiful golden color but also adds anti-inflammatory benefits.

Zucchini Meatballs with Marinara Sauce and Vegan Parmesan

Preparation Time: 25 minutes, **Cooking Time:** 35 minutes, **Servings:** 4

Ingredients:

- For the Zucchini Meatballs:
  - 2 cups grated zucchini (about 2 medium zucchinis)
  - 1 cup breadcrumbs
  - 1/4 cup vegan Parmesan cheese, grated
  - 2 cloves garlic, minced
  - 1 tsp dried oregano
  - 1 tsp dried basil
  - Salt and pepper to taste
  - Olive oil, for cooking
- For the Marinara Sauce:
  - 2 tbsp olive oil
  - 1 onion, finely chopped
  - 2 cloves garlic, minced
  - 1 can (28 oz) crushed tomatoes
  - 1 tsp sugar
  - 1 tbsp dried basil
  - Salt and pepper to taste
- Additional Ingredients:
  - Fresh basil, for garnish and Extra vegan Parmesan cheese, for serving

- Nutritional Values:

Nutrient	Per Serving
Calories	290 kcal
Protein	9 g
Carbohydrates	35 g
Fats	13 g
Dietary Fiber	6 g

Procedure: Preheat the oven to 375°F (190°C).

1. Squeeze the grated zucchini in a clean kitchen towel to remove excess moisture. In a bowl, combine the squeezed zucchini, breadcrumbs, vegan Parmesan, minced garlic, oregano, basil, salt, and pepper. Mix until well combined.

2. Form the mixture into small balls, about the size of a golf ball. Heat a thin layer of olive oil in a skillet over medium heat. Brown the zucchini meatballs on all sides, then transfer them to a baking sheet.

3. Bake in the preheated oven for 20 minutes, until firm and cooked through. For the marinara sauce, heat olive oil in a saucepan over medium heat. Add the onion and garlic, and sauté until soft and translucent. Add the crushed tomatoes, sugar, dried basil, salt, and pepper. Simmer for about 20 minutes to allow the flavors to meld. Serve the baked zucchini meatballs topped with warm marinara sauce, garnished with fresh basil and sprinkled with extra vegan Parmesan.

Metabolism-Friendly Snacks

Celery Sticks with Almond Butter and Honey

Preparation Time: 10 minutes, **Servings:** 4

Ingredients:

- 4 large celery stalks, washed and cut into 3-inch sticks
- 1/2 cup almond butter
- 4 tbsp honey
- Optional toppings: chopped nuts, dried fruit, or a sprinkle of cinnamon

- **Nutritional Values:**

Nutrient	Per Serving
Calories	210 kcal
Protein	4 g
Carbohydrates	20 g
Fats	14 g
Dietary Fiber	3 g

Procedure:

1. Arrange the celery sticks on a serving platter.
2. In a small bowl, mix the almond butter with a little honey to make it easier to spread.
3. Using a knife or a small spoon, fill the celery sticks with the almond butter mixture.
4. Drizzle the remaining honey over the filled celery sticks.
5. If desired, sprinkle with your choice of optional toppings like chopped nuts, dried fruit, or cinnamon for extra flavor and texture.

- **Tips:**
  - For a smoother filling, gently warm the almond butter before mixing with honey.
  - These celery sticks can be made in advance and stored in the refrigerator for a quick snack or appetizer.

Kale Chips with Smoked Paprika and Sea Salt

Preparation Time: 10 minutes, **Cooking Time:** 20 minutes, **Servings:** 4

Ingredients:

- 1 bunch of kale, washed and dried
- 2 tbsp olive oil
- 1 tsp smoked paprika
- Sea salt to taste

Nutritional Values:

Nutrient	Per Serving
Calories	80 kcal
Protein	2 g
Carbohydrates	6 g
Fats	5 g
Dietary Fiber	1 g

Procedure:

5. Preheat your oven to 300°F (150°C).
6. Remove the stems from the kale and tear the leaves into bite-sized pieces.
7. In a large bowl, toss the kale leaves with olive oil until they are evenly coated.
8. Sprinkle the smoked paprika and sea salt over the kale and toss again to distribute the seasonings evenly.
9. Spread the kale in a single layer on a baking sheet lined with parchment paper.
10. Bake in the preheated oven for about 20 minutes, or until the edges are crisp but not burnt, turning halfway through cooking.
11. Let the kale chips cool slightly before serving to allow them to crisp up further.

- Tips:
    - Make sure the kale is thoroughly dry before adding the oil; moisture can prevent the chips from becoming crispy.
    - Keep a close eye on the kale chips, especially towards the end of baking, as they can go from crisp to burnt quickly.

Cauliflower Popcorn with Olive Oil and Vegan Parmesan

Preparation Time: 10 minutes, **Cooking Time:** 25 minutes, **Servings:** 4

Ingredients:

- 1 large head of cauliflower, cut into bite-sized florets
- 3 tbsp olive oil
- 1/2 cup vegan Parmesan cheese, grated
- Salt and pepper to taste

Nutritional Values:

Nutrient	Per Serving
Calories	150 kcal
Protein	5 g
Carbohydrates	10 g
Fats	10 g
Dietary Fiber	3 g

Procedure:

5. Preheat your oven to 400°F (200°C).
6. In a large bowl, toss the cauliflower florets with olive oil until well coated.
7. Sprinkle the vegan Parmesan cheese over the cauliflower, adding salt and pepper to taste, and toss again to evenly coat the florets.
8. Spread the cauliflower in a single layer on a baking sheet lined with parchment paper.
9. Bake in the preheated oven for 20-25 minutes, or until the cauliflower is golden and crispy, stirring halfway through to ensure even cooking.
10. Serve hot, additional vegan Parmesan can be sprinkled on top if desired.

4 Tips:

a. For extra flavor, add a sprinkle of garlic powder or your favorite herbs before baking.
b. Make sure the florets are dry and evenly sized to ensure they crisp up nicely in the oven.

Prosciutto Roll-Ups with Almond Cheese and Green Olives

Preparation Time: 15 minutes, **Servings:** 4

Ingredients:

- 8 slices of prosciutto
- 1/2 cup almond cheese, softened
- 16 green olives, pitted and halved
- Fresh basil leaves (optional)

Nutritional Values:

Nutrient	Per Serving
Calories	180 kcal
Protein	10 g
Carbohydrates	3 g
Fats	14 g
Dietary Fiber	1 g

Procedure:

5. Lay out the slices of prosciutto on a clean surface.
6. Spread a thin layer of almond cheese over each slice of prosciutto.
7. Place a couple of basil leaves (if using) and two halves of green olives at one end of each slice.
8. Carefully roll up the prosciutto around the cheese and olives, starting from the end with the fillings.
9. Secure the roll-ups with toothpicks if necessary.
10. Serve immediately, or chill in the refrigerator for an hour before serving if a firmer texture is desired.

- **Tips:**
    - If almond cheese is too firm to spread, mix it with a little olive oil to soften.
    - These roll-ups can be varied with different fillings such as sun-dried tomatoes, roasted red peppers, or artichoke hearts for different flavors.

Avocado, Spinach, and Green Apple Smoothie

Preparation Time: 10 minutes, **Servings:** 2

Ingredients:

- 1 ripe avocado, peeled and pitted
- 1 green apple, cored and chopped
- 2 cups fresh spinach leaves
- 1 cup unsweetened almond milk
- 1 tablespoon honey or to taste (optional for sweetness)
- Juice of 1/2 lemon
- Ice cubes (optional for a colder smoothie)

- Nutritional Values:

Nutrient	Per Serving
Calories	250 kcal
Protein	3 g
Carbohydrates	27 g
Fats	15 g
Dietary Fiber	7 g

Procedure:

1. Place the avocado, green apple, spinach leaves, almond milk, honey (if using), and lemon juice in a blender.

2. Blend on high until smooth. If the smoothie is too thick, add more almond milk to reach the desired consistency.

3. If a colder smoothie is preferred, add ice cubes and blend again until smooth.

4. Taste and adjust the sweetness with more honey if needed.

5. Serve immediately, pouring into glasses.

- Tips:
  - Adding lemon juice not only enhances the flavor but also helps prevent the avocado from browning.
  - For additional nutrients and a thicker texture, you could add a tablespoon of chia seeds or flaxseeds to the smoothie before blending.

Energy Bites with Dates, Cacao, and Nuts

Preparation Time: 20 minutes, **Chilling Time:** 30 minutes, **Servings:** 12 bites

Ingredients:

- 1 cup dates, pitted
- 1/2 cup raw almonds
- 1/2 cup raw walnuts
- 2 tablespoons cacao powder
- 1 teaspoon vanilla extract
- Pinch of salt
- Optional: shredded coconut or cacao nibs for coating

- Nutritional Values:

Nutrient	Per Serving
Calories	120 kcal
Protein	3 g
Carbohydrates	15 g
Fats	7 g
Dietary Fiber	3 g

Procedure:

1. In a food processor, combine the dates, almonds, and walnuts. Pulse until the mixture is finely chopped and begins to stick together.
2. Add the cacao powder, vanilla extract, and a pinch of salt. Process until the mixture becomes a sticky, uniform dough.
3. Take a tablespoon of the mixture and roll it into a ball. Repeat with the remaining mixture.
4. If desired, roll the energy bites in shredded coconut or cacao nibs to coat.
5. Place the energy bites on a tray and refrigerate for at least 30 minutes to firm up.
6. Store the energy bites in an airtight container in the refrigerator.

- Tips:
  - If the mixture is too dry and not sticking together, you can add a tablespoon of water or a little more vanilla extract to help it bind.
  - These energy bites are highly customizable. Feel free to add other ingredients like chia seeds, flaxseeds, or protein powder for an extra nutritional boost.

Mini Spinach and Mushroom Frittatas

Preparation Time: 15 minutes, **Cooking Time:** 20 minutes, **Servings:** 12 mini frittatas

Ingredients:

- 6 large eggs
- 1 cup fresh spinach, chopped
- 1 cup mushrooms, finely chopped
- 1/2 cup onion, finely chopped
- 1/2 cup grated cheese (optional, can use dairy-free cheese for a vegan version)
- 1/4 cup milk (or non-dairy milk)
- Salt and pepper to taste
- Olive oil or non-stick spray for greasing

- Nutritional Values:

Nutrient	Per Serving
Calories	80 kcal
Protein	6 g
Carbohydrates	2 g
Fats	5 g
Dietary Fiber	0.5 g

- Procedure:

1. Preheat your oven to 375°F (190°C). Grease a 12-cup muffin pan with olive oil or non-stick spray.

2. In a large bowl, beat the eggs and milk together. Add the chopped spinach, mushrooms, onions, and grated cheese. Season with salt and pepper, and mix well.

3. Pour the egg mixture evenly into the muffin cups, filling each about two-thirds full.

4. Bake in the preheated oven for 20 minutes, or until the frittatas are set and the tops are lightly golden.

5. Remove from the oven and let cool for a few minutes before removing from the pan.

6. Serve warm, or let cool completely and store in an airtight container in the refrigerator for up to 4 days.

- Tips:
  - You can add other vegetables like bell peppers or zucchini for extra flavor and nutrients.
  - These mini frittatas are perfect for meal prep and can be reheated quickly for a nutritious breakfast or snack on the go.

Beet Hummus with Vegetable Crudités

Preparation Time: 15 minutes (plus cooking time for beets if using fresh), **Servings:** 4-6

Ingredients:

- **For the Beet Hummus:**
    - 1 large beet (about 1 cup cooked and chopped)
    - 1 can (15 oz) chickpeas, drained and rinsed
    - 2 cloves garlic, minced
    - 2 tbsp tahini
    - Juice of 1 lemon
    - 2 tbsp olive oil
    - Salt and pepper to taste
- **For the Crudités:**
    - A variety of fresh vegetables such as carrots, celery, bell peppers, cucumber, and cherry tomatoes, cut into sticks or slices
- Optional garnishes: chopped parsley, extra olive oil

- **Nutritional Values:**

Nutrient	Per Serving
Calories	180 kcal
Protein	6 g
Carbohydrates	20 g
Fats	9 g
Dietary Fiber	5 g

Procedure:

1. If using fresh beets, wrap the beet in foil and roast in a preheated 400°F (200°C) oven until tender, about 45-60 minutes. Once cooked, peel and chop.

2. In a food processor, combine the cooked beet, chickpeas, garlic, tahini, lemon juice, and olive oil. Blend until smooth. Season with salt and pepper to taste.

3. Transfer the hummus to a serving bowl and drizzle with a little more olive oil, and sprinkle chopped parsley if using.

4. Arrange the sliced vegetables around the bowl of hummus for dipping.

5. Serve immediately or cover and refrigerate until ready to serve.

- **Tips:**
    - For a smoother hummus, peel the chickpeas by gently pinching each one to remove the skin. This step is optional but helps create a creamier texture.
    - Add a splash of cold water to the hummus while blending if it's too thick or if you prefer a lighter consistency.

Toasted Macadamia Nuts with Rosemary and Sea Salt

Preparation Time: 5 minutes, **Cooking Time:** 10 minutes, **Servings:** 4

Ingredients:

- 1 cup macadamia nuts
- 1 tbsp olive oil
- 1 tbsp fresh rosemary, finely chopped
- 1/2 tsp sea salt

- **Nutritional Values:**

Nutrient	Per Serving
Calories	240 kcal
Protein	2 g
Carbohydrates	4 g
Fats	25 g
Dietary Fiber	3 g

Procedure:

1. Preheat your oven to 350°F (175°C).
2. In a bowl, toss the macadamia nuts with olive oil, chopped rosemary, and sea salt until well coated.
3. Spread the nuts in a single layer on a baking sheet lined with parchment paper.
4. Toast in the preheated oven for about 10 minutes, or until golden and fragrant. Be sure to stir the nuts halfway through to ensure even toasting.
5. Remove from the oven and let cool on the baking sheet.
6. Serve as a snack, or use as a topping for salads or other dishes.

- **Tips:**
  - Keep a close eye on the nuts as they toast, as macadamia nuts can burn quickly due to their high-fat content.
  - For extra flavor, you can add a pinch of cracked black pepper or a sprinkle of chili flakes before toasting.

Nori Seaweed Snacks with Avocado and Sesame Seeds

Preparation Time: 10 minutes, **Servings:** 4

Ingredients:
- 4 sheets of nori seaweed
- 1 ripe avocado, mashed
- 1 tbsp sesame seeds (a mix of black and white, if available)
- Optional: a sprinkle of sea salt or a drizzle of soy sauce for extra flavor

- **Nutritional Values:**

Nutrient	Per Serving
Calories	100 kcal
Protein	2 g
Carbohydrates	9 g
Fats	7 g
Dietary Fiber	3 g

Procedure:

1. Lay a sheet of nori on a flat surface.
2. Spread a thin layer of mashed avocado across the nori sheet, leaving a small border around the edges to help seal the roll.
3. Sprinkle sesame seeds evenly over the avocado. If using, add a light sprinkle of sea salt or a light drizzle of soy sauce.
4. Carefully roll the nori sheet tightly from one end to the other. Use a little water along the edge to seal the roll if necessary.
5. Use a sharp knife to slice the roll into bite-sized pieces.
6. Serve immediately, or store in an airtight container.

- **Tips:**
  - Ensure the avocado is ripe enough to spread easily but not too mushy.
  - These snacks are best enjoyed soon after making, as the nori can lose its crispness when exposed to moisture for too long.

Wellness Beverages

Matcha Latte with Almond Milk and Honey

Preparation Time: 5 minutes, **Servings:** 1

Ingredients:

- 1 tsp matcha green tea powder
- 1 cup unsweetened almond milk
- 1 tbsp honey, or to taste
- Hot water (just below boiling point)

- Nutritional Values:

Nutrient	Per Serving
Calories	100 kcal
Protein	2 g
Carbohydrates	19 g
Fats	2.5 g
Dietary Fiber	1 g

Procedure:

1. Sift the matcha green tea powder into a cup to remove any lumps. This ensures a smooth texture in your latte.

2. Add a small amount of hot water (about 2 tablespoons) to the matcha powder. Using a matcha whisk or small regular whisk, stir briskly in a W motion until the tea is frothy and completely dissolved.

3. In a small saucepan, heat the almond milk over medium heat until hot but not boiling. Alternatively, you can use a microwave.

4. Stir the honey into the hot almond milk until fully dissolved.

5. Pour the frothy hot almond milk into the cup with the matcha mixture. Stir gently to combine.

6. If desired, froth the top layer with a milk frother for extra foam.

7. Serve immediately, enjoying the earthy flavors of matcha paired with the subtle sweetness of honey.

- Tips:
    - For a cold version, chill the almond milk and mix all ingredients in a shaker or blender. Serve over ice.
    - Adjust the amount of honey based on your preferred sweetness level.

Iced Lemon Ginger Tea with Fresh Mint

Preparation Time: 10 minutes, **Chilling Time:** 1 hour, **Servings:** 4

Ingredients:

- 4 cups water
- 2 inches fresh ginger, peeled and sliced thinly
- Juice of 2 lemons
- 1/4 cup honey, or to taste
- Fresh mint leaves, for garnish and flavor
- Ice cubes, for serving

- **Nutritional Values:**

Nutrient	Per Serving
Calories	60 kcal
Protein	0 g
Carbohydrates	17 g
Fats	0 g
Dietary Fiber	0 g

Procedure:

1. In a saucepan, bring the water to a boil. Add the sliced ginger and reduce the heat. Let it simmer for about 10 minutes to infuse the water with the ginger.

2. Remove from heat and strain out the ginger pieces. Stir in the honey until dissolved while the tea is still hot.

3. Allow the ginger tea to cool to room temperature. Once cooled, stir in the fresh lemon juice.

4. Refrigerate the tea until chilled, about 1 hour.

5. Serve the iced tea over ice cubes in glasses. Garnish with fresh mint leaves.

6. Optionally, you can add additional lemon slices or a little more honey if a sweeter taste is desired.

- **Tips:**
    - For a stronger mint flavor, you can add mint leaves to the tea while it cools or even while simmering the ginger. This tea can be made in large batches and stored in the refrigerator for up to a week.

Coconut Pineapple Smoothie with Turmeric and Ginger

Preparation Time: 10 minutes, **Servings:** 2

Ingredients:

- 1 cup pineapple chunks, fresh or frozen
- 1 banana, sliced
- 1 cup coconut milk
- 1/2 teaspoon turmeric powder
- 1/2 inch fresh ginger, peeled and grated
- 1 tablespoon honey, or to taste (optional)
- Ice cubes (optional, if using fresh pineapple)

- Nutritional Values:

Nutrient	Per Serving
Calories	250 kcal
Protein	2 g
Carbohydrates	35 g
Fats	12 g
Dietary Fiber	3 g

Procedure:

1. In a blender, combine the pineapple chunks, banana, coconut milk, turmeric powder, and fresh ginger.

2. Blend on high until the mixture is smooth and creamy.

3. Taste the smoothie and add honey if a sweeter flavor is desired. Blend again to incorporate the honey.

4. If the smoothie is too thick or if using fresh pineapple, add ice cubes to achieve the desired consistency and blend again.

5. Pour the smoothie into glasses and serve immediately.

- Tips:
  - If you prefer a colder smoothie and are using fresh pineapple, you can freeze the pineapple chunks prior to blending.
  - Adjust the amount of ginger and turmeric according to your taste preferences; both can be quite potent.

Ginger, Lemon, and Turmeric Herbal Tea

Preparation Time: 5 minutes, **Cooking Time:** 10 minutes, **Servings:** 2

Ingredients:

- 2 cups water
- 1 inch fresh ginger, peeled and sliced
- 1/2 teaspoon turmeric powder or 1-inch fresh turmeric, peeled and sliced
- Juice of 1 lemon
- 1 tablespoon honey (optional)
- A pinch of black pepper (optional, to enhance turmeric absorption)

- Nutritional Values:

Nutrient	Per Serving
Calories	30 kcal
Protein	0 g
Carbohydrates	8 g
Fats	0 g
Dietary Fiber	0 g

Procedure:

1. In a small saucepan, bring the water to a boil. Add the sliced ginger and turmeric to the water.
2. Reduce the heat and let the mixture simmer for about 10 minutes to allow the ginger and turmeric to infuse the water.
3. Remove the saucepan from the heat and strain the tea into cups.
4. Stir in the fresh lemon juice and honey if using.
5. Optionally, add a pinch of black pepper to help with the absorption of turmeric's active compound, curcumin.
6. Serve the tea warm and enjoy its soothing, anti-inflammatory properties.

- Tips:
  - For a stronger flavor, you can increase the amount of ginger or turmeric, or simmer the tea longer.
  - This tea can also be served chilled, making it a refreshing option for warmer days.

Bulletproof Coffee with Coconut Oil and Cinnamon

Preparation Time: 5 minutes, **Servings:** 1

Ingredients:

- 1 cup freshly brewed hot coffee (preferably single-origin, high-quality beans)
- 1 tablespoon coconut oil (or MCT oil)
- 1 tablespoon unsalted butter (or ghee for a lactose-free option)
- A dash of cinnamon (optional)
- Sweetener of choice (optional, such as stevia or honey)

- Nutritional Values:

Nutrient	Per Serving
Calories	220 kcal
Protein	0 g
Carbohydrates	0 g
Fats	24 g
Dietary Fiber	0 g

- **Procedure:**

1. Brew 1 cup of coffee using your preferred method. A French press or pour-over method works well for a richer flavor.
2. Pour the hot coffee into a blender. Add the coconut oil, butter (or ghee), and a dash of cinnamon if using.
3. Blend on high speed for about 30 seconds or until the mixture is smooth and creamy, resembling a frothy latte.
4. Taste and add sweetener if desired, then blend again briefly to mix.
5. Pour the coffee into a mug and enjoy immediately.

- **Tips:**
    - Ensure the coffee is hot to help the fats emulsify smoothly when blended.
    - Bulletproof coffee is designed to be part of a low-carb, high-fat diet and may help with sustained energy and mental clarity.

Chilled Almond Milk with Cocoa and Vanilla

Preparation Time: 5 minutes, **Servings:** 2

Ingredients:

- 2 cups unsweetened almond milk
- 2 tablespoons cocoa powder
- 1 teaspoon vanilla extract
- Sweetener of choice (such as honey, maple syrup, or a sugar substitute), to taste
- Ice cubes (optional)

- **Nutritional Values:**

Nutrient	Per Serving
Calories	60 kcal
Protein	2 g
Carbohydrates	4 g
Fats	4 g
Dietary Fiber	2 g

Procedure:

1. In a blender, combine the almond milk, cocoa powder, vanilla extract, and your chosen sweetener.
2. Blend on high until the cocoa powder is fully incorporated and the mixture is smooth.
3. Taste and adjust sweetness if necessary.
4. Pour the mixture into glasses over ice cubes if a chilled beverage is desired.
5. Serve immediately for a refreshing and chocolaty drink.

- **Tips:**
    - For a richer texture and flavor, you can use a combination of almond milk and coconut milk.
    - This drink can also be heated for a warm, comforting beverage during colder months.

Iced Hibiscus Tea with Lime and Honey

Preparation Time: 10 minutes, **Steeping Time:** 20 minutes, **Servings:** 4

Ingredients:

- 4 cups water
- 1/4 cup dried hibiscus flowers
- Juice of 2 limes
- 2-3 tablespoons honey, or to taste
- Ice cubes
- Lime slices and mint leaves for garnish (optional)

- **Nutritional Values:**

Nutrient	Per Serving
Calories	50 kcal
Protein	0 g
Carbohydrates	13 g
Fats	0 g
Dietary Fiber	0 g

Procedure:

1. In a medium saucepan, bring the water to a boil. Remove from heat and add the dried hibiscus flowers. Cover and let steep for 20 minutes.

2. Strain the mixture into a pitcher, discarding the hibiscus flowers.

3. Stir in the honey and lime juice until the honey is fully dissolved. Adjust the sweetness to taste.

4. Chill the tea in the refrigerator until it is completely cool.

5. Serve over ice, garnished with lime slices and mint leaves if desired.

- **Tips:**
  - Hibiscus tea can be quite tart; start with less honey and add more as needed after tasting.
  - This tea is not only refreshing but also rich in antioxidants and vitamin C, making it a healthy, revitalizing beverage.

Green Smoothie with Kale, Cucumber, and Green Apple

Preparation Time: 10 minutes, **Servings:** 2

Ingredients:

- 2 cups kale, stems removed and leaves roughly chopped
- 1 medium cucumber, peeled and sliced
- 1 green apple, cored and chopped
- Juice of 1 lemon
- 1 cup cold water or coconut water
- Ice cubes (optional for a colder smoothie)
- Optional: 1 tablespoon honey or agave syrup for sweetness

- **Nutritional Values:**

Nutrient	Per Serving
Calories	90 kcal
Protein	2 g
Carbohydrates	21 g
Fats	0.5 g
Dietary Fiber	4 g

Procedure:

1. Place the kale, cucumber, and green apple in a blender.

2. Add the lemon juice and cold water or coconut water. If desired, add honey or agave syrup for a touch of sweetness.

3. Blend on high until all ingredients are thoroughly combined and the smoothie has a smooth, creamy texture.

4. Add ice cubes to the blender and pulse a few more times if a colder consistency is preferred.

5. Serve the smoothie immediately, ensuring it's fresh and vibrant.

- **Tips:**
  - If the smoothie is too thick, add more water or coconut water to achieve your desired consistency.
  - For added nutrition, you can incorporate a tablespoon of chia seeds or a scoop of protein powder before blending.

Chilled Golden Milk with Turmeric and Ginger

Preparation Time: 5 minutes, **Cooking Time:** 10 minutes, **Chilling Time:** 1 hour, **Servings:** 2

Ingredients:

- 2 cups almond milk (or any milk of your choice)
- 1 teaspoon turmeric powder
- 1/2 teaspoon ground ginger
- 1/4 teaspoon black pepper (to enhance turmeric absorption)
- 1 tablespoon honey or maple syrup (adjust to taste)
- 1 cinnamon stick (or 1/2 teaspoon ground cinnamon)
- Optional: 1 teaspoon vanilla extract for added flavor

- **Nutritional Values:**

Nutrient	Per Serving
Calories	80 kcal
Protein	1 g
Carbohydrates	12 g
Fats	3 g
Dietary Fiber	1 g

Procedure:

1. In a small saucepan, combine the almond milk, turmeric powder, ground ginger, black pepper, and cinnamon stick. Heat over medium heat while stirring frequently to prevent the milk from burning.

2. Just before the mixture comes to a boil, reduce the heat and simmer gently for about 10 minutes to allow the flavors to meld together.

3. Remove from heat and stir in the honey or maple syrup, and vanilla extract if using. Adjust sweetness to your liking.

4. Strain the mixture through a fine sieve to remove the cinnamon stick and any large spice particles.

5. Allow the mixture to cool at room temperature before refrigerating until chilled, about 1 hour.

6. Serve the chilled golden milk in glasses, perhaps with an additional sprinkle of cinnamon or turmeric on top for garnish.

- **Tips:**
    - For a creamier texture, consider using coconut milk or a blend of almond and coconut milk.
    - This beverage can also be enjoyed warm, especially during cooler weather, providing a comforting, soothing drink.

Green Juice with Celery, Spinach, and Apple

Preparation Time: 10 minutes, **Servings:** 2

Ingredients:

- 3 stalks celery, chopped
- 2 cups spinach leaves
- 1 green apple, cored and chopped
- 1 cucumber, peeled and chopped
- 1 lemon, peeled and seeded
- 1-inch piece of ginger, peeled
- Optional: a handful of parsley or cilantro for added freshness

- **Nutritional Values:**

Nutrient	Per Serving
Calories	90 kcal
Protein	3 g
Carbohydrates	22 g
Fats	1 g
Dietary Fiber	5 g

Procedure:

1. Wash and prepare all the ingredients by chopping them into smaller pieces as needed.
2. In a juicer, feed the celery, spinach, apple, cucumber, lemon, and ginger, along with any optional herbs, in batches if necessary.
3. Juice until all ingredients are processed and you have a smooth green juice.
4. Stir the juice well and pour into glasses.
5. Serve immediately over ice if desired, ensuring it's fresh and full of nutrients.
6. **Tips:**
    a. Drink the green juice soon after making it to retain the maximum nutrients.
    b. Adjust the sweetness and tanginess by varying the amount of apple and lemon used.

Guilt-Free Desserts

Vegan Lemon Cheesecake with Almond Crust

Preparation Time: 20 minutes, **Chilling Time:** 4 hours, **Servings:** 8

Ingredients:

- For the Almond Crust:
  - 1 1/2 cups almond flour
  - 1/4 cup coconut oil, melted
  - 2 tablespoons maple syrup
  - 1 teaspoon vanilla extract
  - A pinch of salt
- For the Lemon Cheesecake Filling:
  - 1 1/2 cups raw cashews, soaked in water overnight and drained
  - 1/2 cup canned coconut milk, full fat
  - 1/2 cup lemon juice (about 3-4 lemons)
  - 1/3 cup coconut oil, melted
  - 1/2 cup maple syrup
  - Zest of 2 lemons
  - 1 teaspoon vanilla extract

- **Nutritional Values:**

Nutrient	Per Serving
Calories	480 kcal
Protein	10 g
Carbohydrates	34 g
Fats	36 g
Dietary Fiber	4 g

Procedure:

- **For the Crust:** In a mixing bowl, combine almond flour, melted coconut oil, maple syrup, vanilla extract, and a pinch of salt. Mix until well combined and the mixture holds together when pinched.

O. Press the mixture firmly into the bottom of a 9-inch springform pan or pie dish. Set aside in the refrigerator to chill while you make the filling.

- **For the Filling:**

O. In a high-speed blender, combine soaked and drained cashews, coconut milk, lemon juice, melted coconut oil, maple syrup, lemon zest, and vanilla extract. Blend on high until the mixture is completely smooth and creamy. Taste the filling and adjust sweetness or tartness if needed. Pour the filling over the chilled crust and smooth the top with a spatula. Refrigerate for at least 4 hours, or until the cheesecake is firm and set.

Chocolate Mousse with Avocado and Coconut Syrup

Preparation Time: 15 minutes, **Chilling Time:** 1 hour, **Servings:** 4

Ingredients:

- 2 ripe avocados, peeled and pitted
- 1/4 cup raw cacao powder
- 1/4 cup coconut milk
- 1/4 cup coconut syrup (or to taste)
- 1 teaspoon vanilla extract
- Pinch of salt
- Optional toppings: whipped coconut cream, chocolate shavings, or berries

- Nutritional Values:

Nutrient	Per Serving
Calories	250 kcal
Protein	3 g
Carbohydrates	30 g
Fats	15 g
Dietary Fiber	7 g

Procedure:

1. In a blender or food processor, combine the avocados, cacao powder, coconut milk, coconut syrup, vanilla extract, and a pinch of salt.

2. Blend until the mixture is smooth and creamy. Adjust the sweetness by adding more coconut syrup if needed.

3. Divide the mousse into serving dishes and refrigerate for at least 1 hour to set.

4. Before serving, garnish with optional toppings like whipped coconut cream, chocolate shavings, or fresh berries for added flavor and visual appeal.

8 **Tips:**

   a. Ensure the avocados are fully ripe for the best flavor and texture.

   b. For a deeper chocolate taste, you can add a bit more cacao powder or a few drops of chocolate extract.

Paleo Carrot Cake with Coconut Cream

Preparation Time: 20 minutes, **Cooking Time:** 30 minutes, **Servings:** 8

Ingredients:

- For the Cake:
    - 2 cups almond flour
    - 1/2 cup coconut flour
    - 1 teaspoon baking soda
    - 2 teaspoons cinnamon
    - 1/2 teaspoon nutmeg
    - 1/4 teaspoon salt
    - 4 eggs
    - 1/2 cup coconut oil, melted
    - 1/4 cup honey
    - 1 teaspoon vanilla extract
    - 2 cups grated carrots
    - 1/2 cup chopped walnuts (optional)
    - 1/2 cup raisins (optional)
- For the Coconut Cream Frosting:
    - 1 can (14 oz) full-fat coconut milk, chilled overnight
    - 2 tablespoons honey or maple syrup
    - 1 teaspoon vanilla extract

- Nutritional Values:

Nutrient	Per Serving
Calories	360 kcal
Protein	9 g
Carbohydrates	25 g
Fats	25 g
Dietary Fiber	6 g

- Procedure:

1. Preheat your oven to 350°F (175°C). Grease and line an 8-inch cake pan with parchment paper. In a large bowl, mix together the almond flour, coconut flour, baking soda, cinnamon, nutmeg, and salt. In another bowl, whisk together the eggs, melted coconut oil, honey, and vanilla extract until well combined.

2. Stir the wet ingredients into the dry ingredients until just combined. Fold in the grated carrots, walnuts, and raisins if using. Pour the batter into the prepared cake pan and smooth the top with a spatula. Bake in the preheated oven for 30 minutes, or until a toothpick inserted into the center comes out clean.

3. Let the cake cool in the pan for 10 minutes, then turn out onto a wire rack to cool completely. For the frosting, scoop out the solid part of the chilled coconut milk into a bowl (discard the liquid or save for another use). Add honey and vanilla extract, and whip until creamy. Frost the cooled cake with the coconut cream and decorate as desired.

Banana Ice Cream with Pecans and Cacao

Preparation Time: 10 minutes, **Freezing Time:** 2 hours, **Servings:** 4

Ingredients:

- 4 ripe bananas, peeled, sliced, and frozen
- 1/2 cup pecans, toasted and chopped
- 2 tablespoons cacao nibs
- 1 teaspoon vanilla extract
- Optional: 1-2 tablespoons honey or maple syrup for extra sweetness

- **Nutritional Values:**

Nutrient	Per Serving
Calories	220 kcal
Protein	3 g
Carbohydrates	30 g
Fats	10 g
Dietary Fiber	4 g

Procedure:

1. Place the frozen banana slices in a food processor or high-powered blender.

2. Pulse until the bananas break down into small pieces. Continue blending until the mixture becomes creamy and smooth, resembling soft serve ice cream. Scrape down the sides as necessary and add a splash of milk if needed to facilitate blending.

3. Once creamy, add the vanilla extract and optional honey or maple syrup, and blend until combined.

4. Stir in the toasted pecans and cacao nibs by hand or pulse them in gently to distribute evenly.

5. Transfer the ice cream to a container and freeze for at least 2 hours until firm, or enjoy immediately for a softer texture. Serve with additional pecans and cacao nibs sprinkled on top.

- **Tips:**
  - Ensure bananas are very ripe before freezing for the sweetest result.
  - For a smoother texture, occasionally stir the ice cream during the freezing process.

Almond Flour Brownies with Walnuts

Preparation Time: 15 minutes, **Cooking Time:** 25 minutes, **Servings:** 12

Ingredients:

- 1 cup almond flour
- 1/2 cup cocoa powder
- 1/2 teaspoon salt
- 1/2 teaspoon baking soda
- 3 large eggs
- 1/2 cup coconut oil, melted
- 3/4 cup maple syrup or honey
- 1 teaspoon vanilla extract
- 1/2 cup walnuts, chopped
- Optional: 1/2 cup dark chocolate chips

- **Nutritional Values:**

Nutrient	Per Serving
Calories	240 kcal
Protein	5 g
Carbohydrates	18 g
Fats	18 g
Dietary Fiber	3 g

Procedure:

1. Preheat your oven to 350°F (175°C). Grease an 8x8 inch baking dish or line it with parchment paper.
2. In a medium bowl, whisk together almond flour, cocoa powder, salt, and baking soda.
3. In a separate large bowl, mix together eggs, melted coconut oil, maple syrup or honey, and vanilla extract until well combined.
4. Gradually add the dry ingredients to the wet ingredients, stirring until the mixture is smooth.
5. Fold in chopped walnuts and optional chocolate chips.
6. Pour the batter into the prepared baking dish, spreading it evenly.
7. Bake in the preheated oven for 25 minutes, or until a toothpick inserted into the center comes out mostly clean.
8. Let the brownies cool in the pan before cutting into squares.

- **Tips:**
    - For fudgier brownies, reduce the baking time by a few minutes.
    - Allow the brownies to cool completely before cutting to help them set properly and improve texture.

Apple Tartlets with Almond Crust and Cinnamon

Preparation Time: 20 minutes, **Cooking Time:** 25 minutes, **Servings:** 6 tartlets

Ingredients:

- For the Almond Crust:
    - 1 1/2 cups almond flour
    - 2 tablespoons coconut oil, melted
    - 2 tablespoons maple syrup
    - 1 teaspoon vanilla extract
    - A pinch of salt
- For the Apple Filling:
    - 3 medium apples, peeled, cored, and thinly sliced
    - 1 tablespoon coconut oil
    - 1 tablespoon maple syrup
    - 1 teaspoon cinnamon
    - 1/4 teaspoon nutmeg
    - Juice of 1/2 lemon

- Nutritional Values:

Nutrient	Per Serving
Calories	250 kcal
Protein	5 g
Carbohydrates	28 g
Fats	15 g
Dietary Fiber	4 g

Procedure:

1. Preheat your oven to 350°F (175°C). Grease a tartlet pan or line with parchment paper.
2. **For the Crust:**
3. In a bowl, combine almond flour, melted coconut oil, maple syrup, vanilla extract, and a pinch of salt. Stir until the mixture forms a dough. Press the dough evenly into the bottoms and sides of the tartlet pans, ensuring it's compact.
4. Bake the crusts in the preheated oven for 10 minutes, until lightly golden. Remove from the oven and set aside.
5. **For the Apple Filling:**
6. In a skillet, melt the coconut oil over medium heat. Add the sliced apples, maple syrup, cinnamon, nutmeg, and lemon juice. Cook for about 5-7 minutes, stirring occasionally, until the apples are soft and caramelized.
7. Spoon the apple filling evenly into the pre-baked almond crusts.
8. Return the tartlets to the oven and bake for an additional 10-15 minutes, until the apples are tender and the crust is golden brown. Let the tartlets cool slightly before removing from the pan. Serve warm or at room temperature.

Oatmeal Blueberry Cookies with Coconut Flour

Preparation Time: 15 minutes, **Cooking Time:** 12-15 minutes, **Servings:** 12 cookies

Ingredients:

- 1 cup rolled oats
- 1/2 cup coconut flour
- 1/2 teaspoon baking soda
- 1/4 teaspoon salt
- 1/4 cup coconut oil, melted
- 1/4 cup honey or maple syrup
- 1 teaspoon vanilla extract
- 1 egg (or flax egg for vegan option)
- 1/2 cup fresh or frozen blueberries

- **Nutritional Values:**

Nutrient	Per Serving
Calories	120 kcal
Protein	3 g
Carbohydrates	18 g
Fats	5 g
Dietary Fiber	3 g

Procedure:

1. Preheat your oven to 350°F (175°C). Line a baking sheet with parchment paper.
2. In a large bowl, combine the rolled oats, coconut flour, baking soda, and salt.
3. In another bowl, whisk together the melted coconut oil, honey (or maple syrup), vanilla extract, and egg until well combined.
4. Stir the wet ingredients into the dry ingredients until a dough forms. Gently fold in the blueberries.
5. Using a tablespoon, drop rounded portions of the dough onto the prepared baking sheet, flattening them slightly.
6. Bake for 12-15 minutes, or until the edges are golden brown.
7. Allow the cookies to cool on the baking sheet for 5 minutes before transferring them to a wire rack to cool completely.

- **Tips:**
  - If using frozen blueberries, do not thaw them before adding to the dough to prevent excess moisture.
  - For a twist, add a handful of chopped nuts or seeds to the cookie dough.

Coconut Lime Mousse with Ginger

Preparation Time: 15 minutes, **Chilling Time:** 2 hours, **Servings:** 4

Ingredients:

- 1 can (14 oz) full-fat coconut milk, chilled overnight
- 1/4 cup lime juice (about 2 limes)
- Zest of 2 limes
- 2 tablespoons honey or maple syrup (adjust to taste)
- 1 teaspoon fresh ginger, grated
- 1/2 teaspoon vanilla extract
- Optional toppings: shredded coconut, lime zest, or fresh berries

- **Nutritional Values:**

Nutrient	Per Serving
Calories	250 kcal
Protein	2 g
Carbohydrates	15 g
Fats	22 g
Dietary Fiber	2 g

Procedure:

1. Scoop the solid part of the chilled coconut milk into a mixing bowl, leaving the liquid behind.

2. Using an electric mixer, whip the coconut cream on high speed for 2-3 minutes until light and fluffy.

3. Add the lime juice, lime zest, honey or maple syrup, grated ginger, and vanilla extract. Continue whipping until everything is well incorporated and the mixture is creamy.

4. Taste the mousse and adjust sweetness if necessary.

5. Spoon the mousse into serving glasses or bowls and refrigerate for at least 2 hours to allow the flavors to meld and the mousse to firm up.

6. Before serving, garnish with optional toppings such as shredded coconut, extra lime zest, or fresh berries.

- **Tips:**
  - Make sure to use full-fat coconut milk and chill it overnight to ensure the cream separates from the liquid.
  - This mousse can also be used as a filling for a tart or pie crust.

Dark Chocolate Truffles with Chili Pepper

Preparation Time: 20 minutes, **Chilling Time:** 2 hours, **Servings:** 16 truffles

Ingredients:

- 8 oz dark chocolate (70% cacao or higher), finely chopped
- 1/2 cup coconut cream (from a chilled can of full-fat coconut milk)
- 1 tablespoon coconut oil
- 1/2 teaspoon ground chili pepper (adjust to taste)
- 1/2 teaspoon vanilla extract
- Optional: cocoa powder or shredded coconut for coating

- Nutritional Values:

Nutrient	Per Serving
Calories	120 kcal
Protein	1 g
Carbohydrates	8 g
Fats	10 g
Dietary Fiber	2 g

Procedure:

1. In a small saucepan, heat the coconut cream and coconut oil over low heat until just simmering. Remove from heat.

2. Add the finely chopped dark chocolate to the saucepan and let it sit for 1-2 minutes to melt. Stir gently until smooth and fully melted.

3. Stir in the ground chili pepper and vanilla extract, mixing until well combined. Adjust the level of spice to your taste.

4. Pour the chocolate mixture into a bowl and refrigerate for about 2 hours, or until the mixture is firm enough to roll.

5. Once firm, scoop out small portions of the chocolate mixture using a spoon or a melon baller, and roll them into balls with your hands.

6. Roll each truffle in cocoa powder or shredded coconut to coat.

7. Store the truffles in the refrigerator until ready to serve.

- Tips:
    - The chili pepper adds a subtle heat that complements the richness of the dark chocolate, but you can adjust the amount based on your spice tolerance.
    - For extra texture, you can add finely chopped nuts to the truffle mixture before chilling.

Pumpkin Pie with Nut Crust and Maple Syrup

Preparation Time: 20 minutes, **Cooking Time:** 50 minutes, **Servings:** 8

Ingredients:

- For the Nut Crust:
    - 1 1/2 cups mixed nuts (almonds, pecans, or walnuts)
    - 2 tablespoons coconut oil, melted
    - 2 tablespoons maple syrup
    - 1 teaspoon cinnamon
    - A pinch of salt
- For the Pumpkin Filling:
    - 1 1/2 cups pumpkin puree (canned or homemade)
    - 1/2 cup coconut milk
    - 1/3 cup maple syrup
    - 2 large eggs
    - 1 teaspoon vanilla extract
    - 1 teaspoon cinnamon
    - 1/2 teaspoon ground ginger
    - 1/4 teaspoon ground nutmeg
    - 1/4 teaspoon ground cloves
    - A pinch of salt

- Nutritional Values:

Nutrient	Per Serving
Calories	290 kcal
Protein	5 g
Carbohydrates	25 g
Fats	20 g
Dietary Fiber	4 g

- Procedure:

1. Preheat your oven to 350°F (175°C). Grease a 9-inch pie dish.

2. **For the Nut Crust:** In a food processor, pulse the mixed nuts until finely ground, but not too powdery. In a bowl, mix the ground nuts, melted coconut oil, maple syrup, cinnamon, and a pinch of salt until combined. Press the mixture firmly into the bottom and up the sides of the pie dish to form the crust. Bake for 10 minutes, then remove from the oven and set aside.

3. **For the Pumpkin Filling:** In a large bowl, whisk together the pumpkin puree, coconut milk, maple syrup, eggs, vanilla extract, spices, and salt until smooth. Pour the filling into the pre-baked nut crust.

4. Bake the pie for 40-45 minutes, or until the filling is set and a toothpick inserted into the center comes out clean. Let the pie cool completely before slicing. Serve with a dollop of coconut whipped cream or a drizzle of maple syrup if desired.

Special Occasion Recipes

Quinoa Paella with Shrimp and Vegetables

Preparation Time: 20 minutes, **Cooking Time:** 30 minutes, **Servings:** 4

Ingredients:

- 1 cup quinoa, rinsed
- 2 cups vegetable or chicken broth
- 1 lb shrimp, peeled and deveined
- 1 tablespoon olive oil
- 1 onion, finely chopped
- 3 cloves garlic, minced
- 1 bell pepper, sliced
- 1 zucchini, sliced
- 1/2 cup peas (fresh or frozen)
- 1 teaspoon smoked paprika
- 1/4 teaspoon saffron threads
- 1 teaspoon turmeric
- Salt and pepper to taste
- Fresh parsley, chopped, for garnish
- Lemon wedges, for serving

- **Nutritional Values:**

Nutrient	Per Serving
Calories	400 kcal
Protein	30 g
Carbohydrates	45 g
Fats	10 g
Dietary Fiber	6 g

Procedure:

1. **For the Quinoa:** In a medium saucepan, bring the vegetable or chicken broth to a boil. Add the rinsed quinoa, cover, and reduce the heat to low. Simmer for about 15 minutes, or until the quinoa is cooked and the liquid is absorbed. Fluff with a fork and set aside.

2. **For the Shrimp and Vegetables:** In a large skillet or paella pan, heat the olive oil over medium heat. Add the chopped onion and garlic and sauté for 2-3 minutes until softened. Add the bell pepper, zucchini, and peas, cooking for 5-7 minutes until the vegetables are tender but still crisp. Stir in the smoked paprika, saffron threads (if using), and turmeric

3. **For the Shrimp:** Push the vegetables to the side of the skillet and add the shrimp. Cook for 2-3 minutes on each side until the shrimp are pink and opaque. Season with salt and pepper to taste.

4. **To Assemble the Paella:** Stir the cooked quinoa into the skillet with the shrimp and vegetables, mixing everything together. Allow the paella to cook for another 5 minutes, letting the flavors combine. **To Serve:** Garnish with fresh parsley and serve with lemon wedges on the side for an extra burst of flavor.

Zucchini Lasagna with Vegan Ricotta and Spinach

Preparation Time: 30 minutes, **Cooking Time:** 45 minutes, **Servings:** 6

Ingredients:

- For the Zucchini "Noodles":
    - 4 large zucchinis, sliced lengthwise into thin strips
    - 1 tablespoon olive oil
    - Salt and pepper to taste
- For the Vegan Ricotta:
    - 1 1/2 cups raw cashews, soaked for at least 4 hours or overnight, drained
    - 1/4 cup nutritional yeast
    - 2 tablespoons lemon juice
    - 1 clove garlic, minced
    - 1/4 cup unsweetened almond milk (or other non-dairy milk)
    - Salt and pepper to taste
- For the Spinach Layer:
    - 2 cups fresh spinach, chopped
    - 1 tablespoon olive oil
    - 1 clove garlic, minced
- For the Tomato Sauce:
    - 2 cups marinara sauce (store-bought or homemade)
    - 1 teaspoon dried oregano
    - 1 teaspoon dried basil
- Optional toppings: fresh basil, vegan Parmesan, or crushed red pepper flakes

- Nutritional Values:

Nutrient	Per Serving
Calories	350 kcal
Protein	10 g
Carbohydrates	18 g
Fats	28 g
Dietary Fiber	5 g

- Procedure:

1. For the Zucchini "Noodles":
    - Preheat the oven to 375°F (190°C). Lightly salt the zucchini slices and let them sit for 10 minutes to draw out excess moisture. Pat them dry with a paper towel.

- Brush the zucchini slices with olive oil and season with salt and pepper. Set aside.

2. **For the Vegan Ricotta:**
    - In a food processor, combine the soaked cashews, nutritional yeast, lemon juice, garlic, almond milk, salt, and pepper. Process until smooth and creamy, adding more almond milk if needed for a spreadable consistency.

3. **For the Spinach Layer:**
    - In a skillet, heat 1 tablespoon of olive oil over medium heat. Add the garlic and sauté for 1 minute, then add the chopped spinach. Cook until the spinach wilts, about 3-4 minutes. Set aside.

4. **To Assemble the Lasagna:**
    - In a baking dish, spread a thin layer of marinara sauce. Lay zucchini slices over the sauce to create the first layer.
    - Spread half of the vegan ricotta over the zucchini, followed by half of the sautéed spinach. Add another layer of marinara sauce.
    - Repeat with another layer of zucchini slices, vegan ricotta, spinach, and sauce, finishing with a layer of zucchini on top.

5. Bake for 40-45 minutes, or until the zucchini is tender and the top is golden. Let it sit for 10 minutes before serving.

6. Garnish with fresh basil, vegan Parmesan, or crushed red pepper flakes if desired.

Baked Chicken with Walnut Sauce and Roasted Broccoli

Preparation Time: 15 minutes, **Cooking Time:** 35 minutes, **Servings:** 4

Ingredients:

- For the Baked Chicken:
    - 4 boneless, skinless chicken breasts
    - 2 tablespoons olive oil
    - 1 teaspoon garlic powder
    - 1 teaspoon paprika
    - Salt and pepper to taste
- For the Walnut Sauce:
    - 1 cup walnuts, toasted
    - 1/2 cup unsweetened almond milk (or other non-dairy milk)
    - 1 tablespoon lemon juice
    - 1 clove garlic, minced
    - 2 tablespoons olive oil
    - Salt and pepper to taste
- For the Roasted Broccoli:
    - 4 cups broccoli florets
    - 2 tablespoons olive oil
    - 1 teaspoon garlic powder
    - Salt and pepper to taste
- Optional garnish: fresh parsley or extra toasted walnuts

- Nutritional Values:

Nutrient	Per Serving
Calories	450 kcal
Protein	35 g
Carbohydrates	10 g
Fats	30 g
Dietary Fiber	5 g

Procedure:

1. **For the Chicken:** Preheat your oven to 375°F (190°C). Rub the chicken breasts with olive oil, garlic powder, paprika, salt, and pepper. Place the chicken on a baking sheet and bake for 25-30 minutes, or until the internal temperature reaches 165°F (74°C).

2. **For the Roasted Broccoli:** While the chicken is baking, toss the broccoli florets with olive oil, garlic powder, salt, and pepper. Spread the broccoli on a separate baking sheet and roast in the oven for 20-25 minutes, or until tender and slightly crispy at the edges.

3. **For the Walnut Sauce:** In a blender or food processor, combine the toasted walnuts, almond milk, lemon juice, garlic, olive oil, salt, and pepper. Blend until smooth and creamy. Add more almond milk if necessary to reach the desired consistency. **To Serve:** Once the chicken is done, plate it alongside the roasted broccoli.

Sweet Potato Gnocchi with Mushroom Sage Sauce

Preparation Time: 30 minutes, **Cooking Time:** 20 minutes, **Servings:** 4

Ingredients:

- 2 large sweet potatoes (about 1 1/2 cups mashed)
- 1 cup almond flour
- 1/2 cup tapioca flour (plus more for dusting)
- 1/2 teaspoon salt
- 2 tablespoons olive oil or vegan butter
- 2 cups mushrooms, sliced (such as cremini or shiitake)
- 1 clove garlic, minced
- 1/4 cup vegetable broth
- 1/2 cup coconut milk or almond milk
- 1 tablespoon fresh sage, finely chopped (or 1 teaspoon dried sage)
- Salt and pepper to taste
  - Optional garnish: fresh sage leaves or grated vegan Parmesan

- **Nutritional Values:**

Nutrient	Per Serving
Calories	350 kcal
Protein	6 g
Carbohydrates	45 g
Fats	15 g
Dietary Fiber	7 g

Procedure:

1. **For the Sweet Potato Gnocchi:** Preheat the oven to 400°F (200°C). Roast the sweet potatoes in the oven for 45-50 minutes, or until soft. Once cooked, scoop out the flesh and mash until smooth. In a large bowl, combine the mashed sweet potatoes, almond flour, tapioca flour, and salt. Mix until a dough forms. If the dough is too sticky, add more tapioca flour, 1 tablespoon at a time. Divide the dough into 4 portions. Roll each portion into a long rope about 1 inch thick. Cut the rope into small gnocchi pieces and dust with extra tapioca flour to prevent sticking.

2. **To Cook the Gnocchi:** Bring a large pot of salted water to a boil. Add the gnocchi in batches and cook for about 3-4 minutes, or until they float to the surface. Remove with a slotted spoon and set aside.

3. **For the Mushroom Sage Sauce:** In a large skillet, heat olive oil or vegan butter over medium heat. Add the sliced mushrooms and cook until browned and softened, about 5-7 minutes. Add the minced garlic and cook for another 1-2 minutes until fragrant. Stir in the vegetable broth, coconut milk, and chopped sage. Simmer for 5 minutes, allowing the sauce to thicken slightly. Season with salt and pepper to taste.

4. **To Serve:** Toss the cooked gnocchi in the mushroom sage sauce.

Lettuce Tacos with Bison Meat and Avocado Salsa

Preparation Time: 20 minutes, **Cooking Time:** 15 minutes, **Servings:** 4

Ingredients:

- For the Bison Meat:
  - 1 lb ground bison
  - 1 tablespoon olive oil
  - 1 small onion, finely chopped
  - 2 cloves garlic, minced
  - 1 teaspoon cumin
  - 1 teaspoon smoked paprika
  - 1/2 teaspoon chili powder
  - Salt and pepper to taste
- For the Avocado Salsa:
  - 2 ripe avocados, diced
  - 1 small tomato, diced
  - 1/4 cup red onion, finely chopped
  - Juice of 1 lime
  - 2 tablespoons fresh cilantro, chopped
  - Salt and pepper to taste
- For the Lettuce Tacos:
  - 8 large lettuce leaves (such as romaine or butter lettuce)
  - Optional toppings: chopped cilantro, sliced jalapeños, or hot sauce

- Nutritional Values:

Nutrient	Per Serving
Calories	350 kcal
Protein	24 g
Carbohydrates	12 g
Fats	25 g
Dietary Fiber	7 g

- Procedure:

1. **For the Bison Meat:** In a large skillet, heat olive oil over medium heat. Add the chopped onion and garlic and sauté until softened, about 3 minutes. Add the ground bison to the skillet, breaking it up with a spoon as it cooks. Cook until browned, about 5-7 minutes. Stir in the cumin, smoked paprika, chili powder, salt, and pepper. Cook for another 2 minutes, allowing the spices to infuse the meat. Remove from heat.

2. **For the Avocado Salsa:** In a bowl, combine the diced avocados, tomato, red onion, lime juice, chopped cilantro, salt, and pepper. Gently toss to mix the ingredients.

3. **To Assemble the Lettuce Tacos:** Lay the lettuce leaves flat on a serving platter. Spoon the cooked bison mixture onto each lettuce leaf. Top each taco with a generous serving of avocado salsa. Garnish with optional toppings like chopped cilantro, sliced jalapeños, or a drizzle of hot sauce. Serve immediately and enjoy!

Quinoa Paella with Shrimp and Vegetables

Preparation Time: 20 minutes, **Cooking Time:** 30 minutes, **Servings:** 4

Ingredients:

- 1 cup quinoa, rinsed
- 2 cups vegetable or chicken broth
- 1 lb shrimp, peeled and deveined
- 1 tablespoon olive oil
- 1 onion, finely chopped
- 3 cloves garlic, minced
- 1 bell pepper, sliced
- 1 zucchini, sliced
- 1/2 cup peas (fresh or frozen)
- 1 teaspoon smoked paprika
- 1/4 teaspoon saffron threads (optional, for authentic flavor)
- 1 teaspoon turmeric
- Salt and pepper to taste
- Fresh parsley, chopped, for garnish
- Lemon wedges, for serving

- **Nutritional Values:**

Nutrient	Per Serving
Calories	400 kcal
Protein	30 g
Carbohydrates	45 g
Fats	10 g
Dietary Fiber	6 g

Procedure:

1. **For the Quinoa:** In a medium saucepan, bring the vegetable or chicken broth to a boil. Add the rinsed quinoa, cover, and reduce the heat to low. Simmer for about 15 minutes, or until the quinoa is cooked and the liquid is absorbed. Fluff with a fork and set aside.

2. **For the Shrimp and Vegetables:** In a large skillet or paella pan, heat the olive oil over medium heat. Add the chopped onion and garlic and sauté for 2-3 minutes until softened. Add the bell pepper, zucchini, and peas, cooking for 5-7 minutes until the vegetables are tender but still crisp. Stir in the smoked paprika, saffron threads (if using), and turmeric. Cook for another minute until fragrant.

3. **For the Shrimp:** Push the vegetables to the side of the skillet and add the shrimp. Cook for 2-3 minutes on each side until the shrimp are pink and opaque. Season with salt and pepper to taste.

4. **To Assemble the Paella:** Stir the cooked quinoa into the skillet with the shrimp and vegetables, mixing everything together. Allow the paella to cook for another 5 minutes, letting the flavors combine.

5. **To Serve:** Garnish with fresh parsley and serve with lemon wedges on the side for an extra burst of flavor.

Mediterranean Vegetable Stew with Olives and Capers

Preparation Time: 15 minutes, **Cooking Time:** 40 minutes, **Servings:** 4

Ingredients:

- 2 tablespoons olive oil
- 1 onion, finely chopped
- 2 cloves garlic, minced
- 1 large eggplant, diced
- 1 zucchini, diced
- 1 red bell pepper, diced
- 1 yellow bell pepper, diced
- 1 can (14 oz) diced tomatoes
- 1/2 cup vegetable broth
- 1/4 cup green or black olives, pitted and halved
- 2 tablespoons capers, drained
- 1 teaspoon dried oregano
- 1 teaspoon dried thyme
- Salt and pepper to taste
- Fresh parsley or basil, chopped, for garnish
- Optional: crusty bread or cooked quinoa for serving

- **Nutritional Values:**

Nutrient	Per Serving
Calories	280 kcal
Protein	5 g
Carbohydrates	30 g
Fats	16 g
Dietary Fiber	8 g

Procedure:

1. **For the Stew Base:** In a large pot, heat the olive oil over medium heat. Add the chopped onion and garlic, sautéing for 3-4 minutes until softened and fragrant. Add the diced eggplant, zucchini, and bell peppers to the pot. Cook for 8-10 minutes, stirring occasionally, until the vegetables begin to soften and brown slightly.

2. **For the Tomato Broth:** Stir in the diced tomatoes, vegetable broth, oregano, thyme, salt, and pepper. Bring the mixture to a simmer, then reduce the heat to low. Cover the pot and let the stew simmer for 20-25 minutes, stirring occasionally, until the vegetables are tender.

3. **For the Olives and Capers:** Once the vegetables are tender, stir in the olives and capers. Simmer for an additional 5 minutes to allow the flavors to meld together.

4. **To Serve:** Taste and adjust seasoning if needed. Serve the Mediterranean vegetable stew garnished with fresh parsley or basil. Pair it with crusty bread or quinoa for a complete meal.

Chicken Fajitas with Peppers and Cilantro Salsa

Preparation Time: 20 minutes, **Cooking Time:** 15 minutes, **Servings:** 4

Ingredients:

- For the Chicken Fajitas:
    - 1 lb boneless, skinless chicken breasts, sliced into thin strips
    - 2 tablespoons olive oil
    - 1 red bell pepper, sliced
    - 1 yellow bell pepper, sliced
    - 1 onion, sliced
    - 2 cloves garlic, minced
    - 1 teaspoon cumin
    - 1 teaspoon smoked paprika
    - 1/2 teaspoon chili powder
    - Salt and pepper to taste
    - 8 small tortillas (corn or flour)
- For the Cilantro Salsa:
    - 1/2 cup fresh cilantro, chopped
    - 1 small tomato, diced
    - 1/4 cup red onion, finely chopped
    - Juice of 1 lime
    - Salt and pepper to taste
- Optional toppings: avocado slices, sour cream, grated cheese, or hot sauce

- **Nutritional Values:**

Nutrient	Per Serving
Calories	350 kcal
Protein	30 g
Carbohydrates	35 g
Fats	12 g
Dietary Fiber	5 g

Procedure:

1. **For the Chicken Fajitas:** In a large skillet, heat 1 tablespoon of olive oil over medium heat. Add the sliced chicken and season with cumin, smoked paprika, chili powder, salt, and pepper. Cook for about 5-7 minutes until the chicken is browned and cooked through. Remove from the skillet and set aside. In the same skillet, add the remaining olive oil. Add the sliced bell peppers, onion, and garlic, and cook for about 5 minutes, or until the vegetables are tender and slightly charred. Return the cooked chicken to the skillet and toss with the vegetables. Squeeze lime juice over the fajitas and remove from heat.

2. **For the Cilantro Salsa:** In a small bowl, combine the chopped cilantro, diced tomato, red onion, lime juice, salt, and pepper. Stir until well mixed and set aside to serve fresh with the fajitas. **To Serve:** Warm the tortillas in a dry skillet or microwave. Assemble the fajitas by filling each tortilla with the chicken and pepper mixture, then topping with the cilantro salsa.

BONUS WITH QR CODE

Scan it to download 3 EXCLUSIVE BONUS